European School of Oncology

Intercity Report

Series Editor: U. Veronesi

S. Monfardini (Ed.)

The Management of Non-Hodgkin's Lymphomas in Europe

With 13 Figures and 12 Tables

Springer-Verlag Berlin Heidelberg New York
London Paris Tokyo Hong Kong Barcelona

Contents

Management of Non-Hodgkin's Lymphomas in Europe

Silvio Monfardini

Division of Medical Oncology, Centro di Riferimento Oncologico, Aviano, Italy

This report originated in the work of four Intercity Meetings held in different geographical areas of Europe from December 1986 to June 1988. Current strategies of treatment were discussed with varying emphasis on the main clinical situations. Each successive meeting reflected many different points of view, but also variations in attitude due to new information becoming available for some of the later meetings. Since the main contribution to these initiatives was that of medical oncologists and haematologists, a further effort has been required in this report to consider other aspects such as those related to the epidemiological dimensions of the problem, pathology, radiotherapy, treatment of paediatric cases. Moreover, treatment of elderly patients and of patients with HIV infection has received special attention

Despite the attempt to cover several different issues, this report was not intended to be comprehensive, but rather to serve as an assessment of the work which is being conducted in the field of non-Hodgkin's lymphomas in various areas of Europe. The reader will thus have the opportunity of verifying the overall situation with regard to treatment and results achieved in the last five years in Europe.

Epidemiology of Non-Hodgkin's Lymphomas in Europe

Silvia Franceschi

Epidemiology Unit, Centro di Riferimento Oncologico, Aviano, Italy

Non-Hodgkin's lymphoma (NHL) is recognised as a heterogeneous group of disorders resulting from the malignant transformation of lymphoid cells [1]. Until recently, the various pathological classifications of NHL have been a continuing source of confusion. In 1982, the Working Formulation of the Non-Hodgkin's Lymphomas for Clinical Usage was published [2]. This is a clinico-pathological classification that enables translation among the six major existing systems of classifying NHL. More recently, advances in monoclonal antibody studies and cytochemical techniques [3] have enabled an even more precise definition of cell populations involved in NHL. Newer classifications, however, are being very slowly incorporated in epidemiological studies, particularly in descriptive epidemiology ones, which generally employ the criteria of the 9th Revision of the International Classification of Diseases (ICD) [4]. Furthermore, mistakes probably persist even within this limited classification (e.g., confusion between Hodgkin's Disease and NHL), especially in large investigations conducted in less developed countries and in older age groups [5]. Bearing these limitations in mind, this chapter examines the present knowledge on the epidemiology of NHL, with special reference to data from European and, particularly, Italian sources.

Descriptive Epidemiology

Geographical Trends

Knowledge of changing trends in lymphoma incidence and mortality, whether geographical or temporal, is of interest since it may provide important insights into the aetiology and the value of new treatments of these malignancies. Figure 1 shows the world-population standardised incidence rates of NHL from all the European areas covered by Cancer Registries, as they were published in the latest volume of Cancer Incidence in Five Continents [6]. It refers only to the major ICD categories 200 (lymphosarcoma and reticulosarcoma) and 202 (other malignant neoplasms of lymphoid and histiocytic tissue) and shows broad variations, notably in males. The highest-risk areas (e.g., Switzerland, Vaud) have incidence rates approximately five times more elevated than the lowest-risk areas (e.g., Hungary, Vas). Wide variations in registration procedures and in the quality certification/verification of NHL cases can, however, heavily distort international comparisons and it is, to this extent, notable that the highest incidence rates are invariably found in rich, industrialised countries, whereas relatively low rates were reported in East-European countries. However, when 35-64 truncated incidence rates are considered, in order to discount the broader variation in diagnostic standards in the elderly, the range of NHL incidence rates does not become substantially narrower and the ranks of various countries tend to remain the same (Fig. 2). Turning to Cancer Registries outside Europe [6], the most striking feature is the extent to which the age distribution of NHL varies geographically: in rich countries risk for NHL increases with age after adolescence, while in poor countries NHL is more common in children. Notably, in the only African Cancer Registry (Ibadan, Nigeria) [7] a very high incidence of NHL is reported (18% of all tumours), deriving from the very high incidence of Burkitt's lymphoma in malaria-endemic areas.

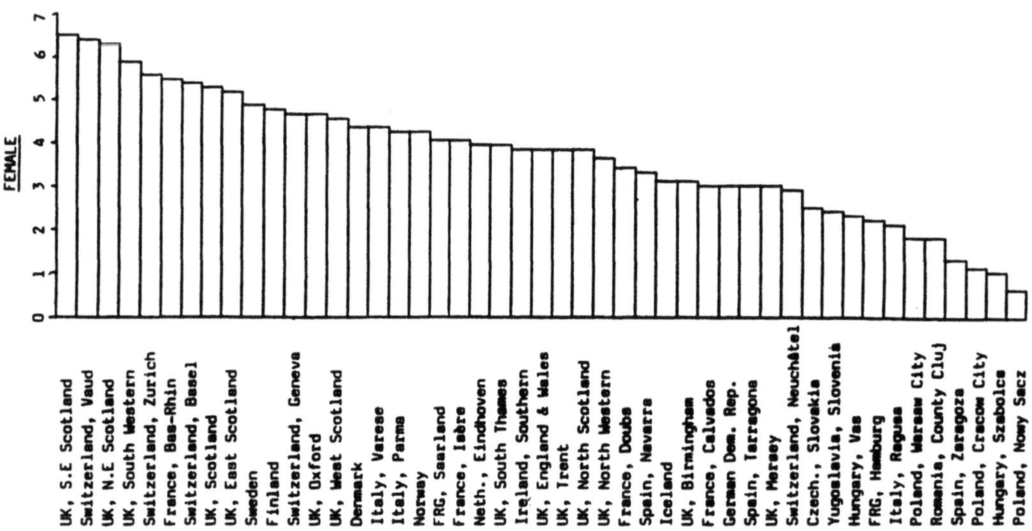

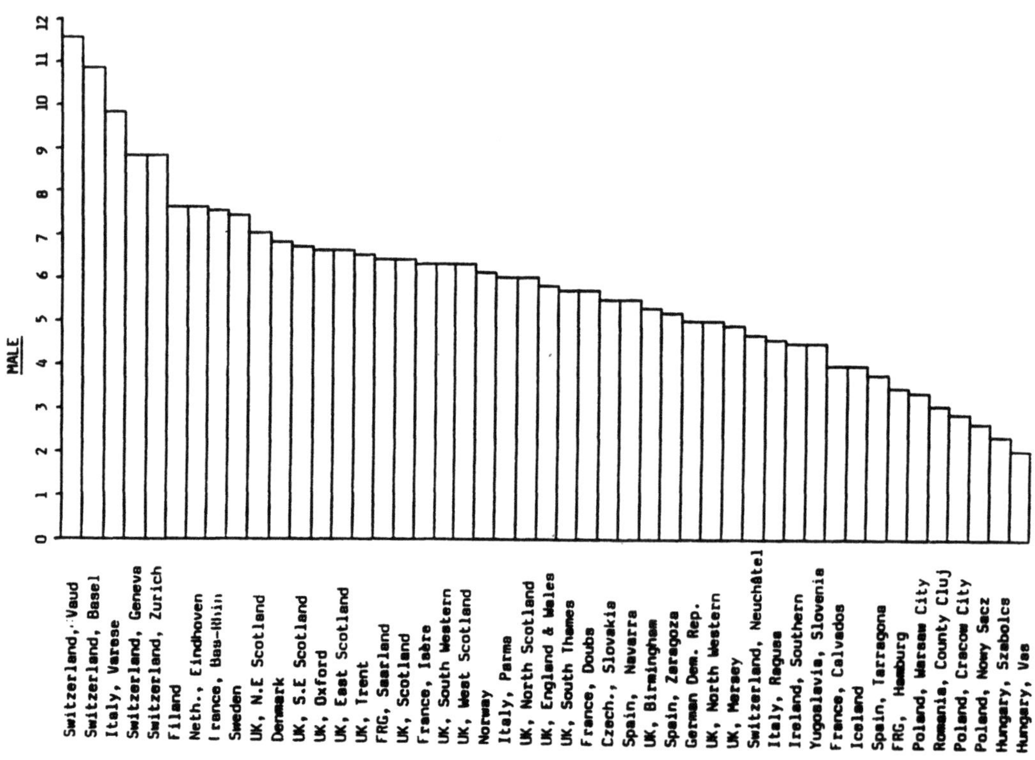

Fig. 1. Average age-standardised incidence rates per 100,000 of non-Hodgkin's lymphoma (ICD-9 200 and 202) in European cancer registries (1978-1982) [6]

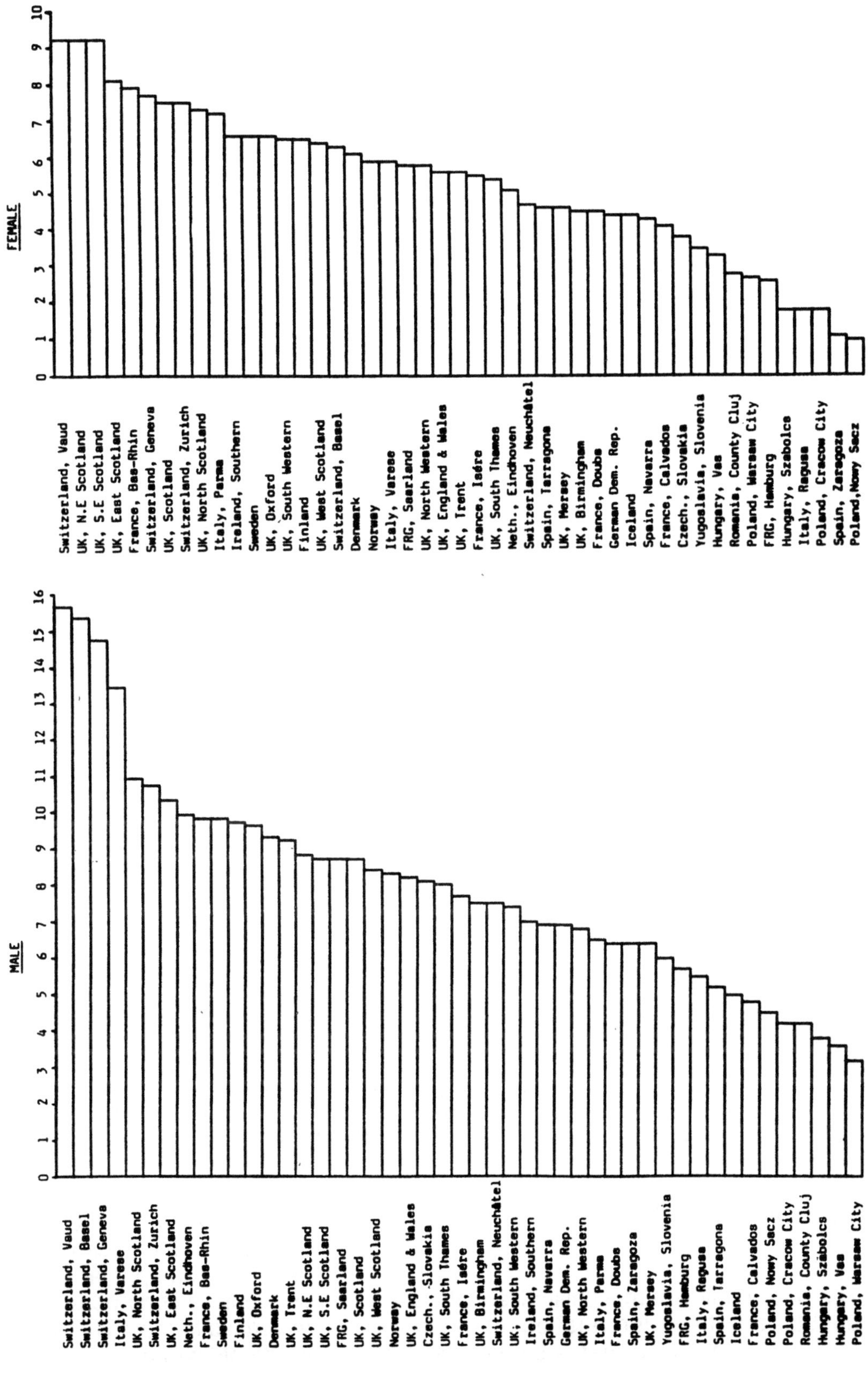

Fig. 2. Average (35-64) truncated incidence rates of non-Hodgkin's lymphoma (ICD9 200 and 202) in European cancer registries (1978-1982) [6]

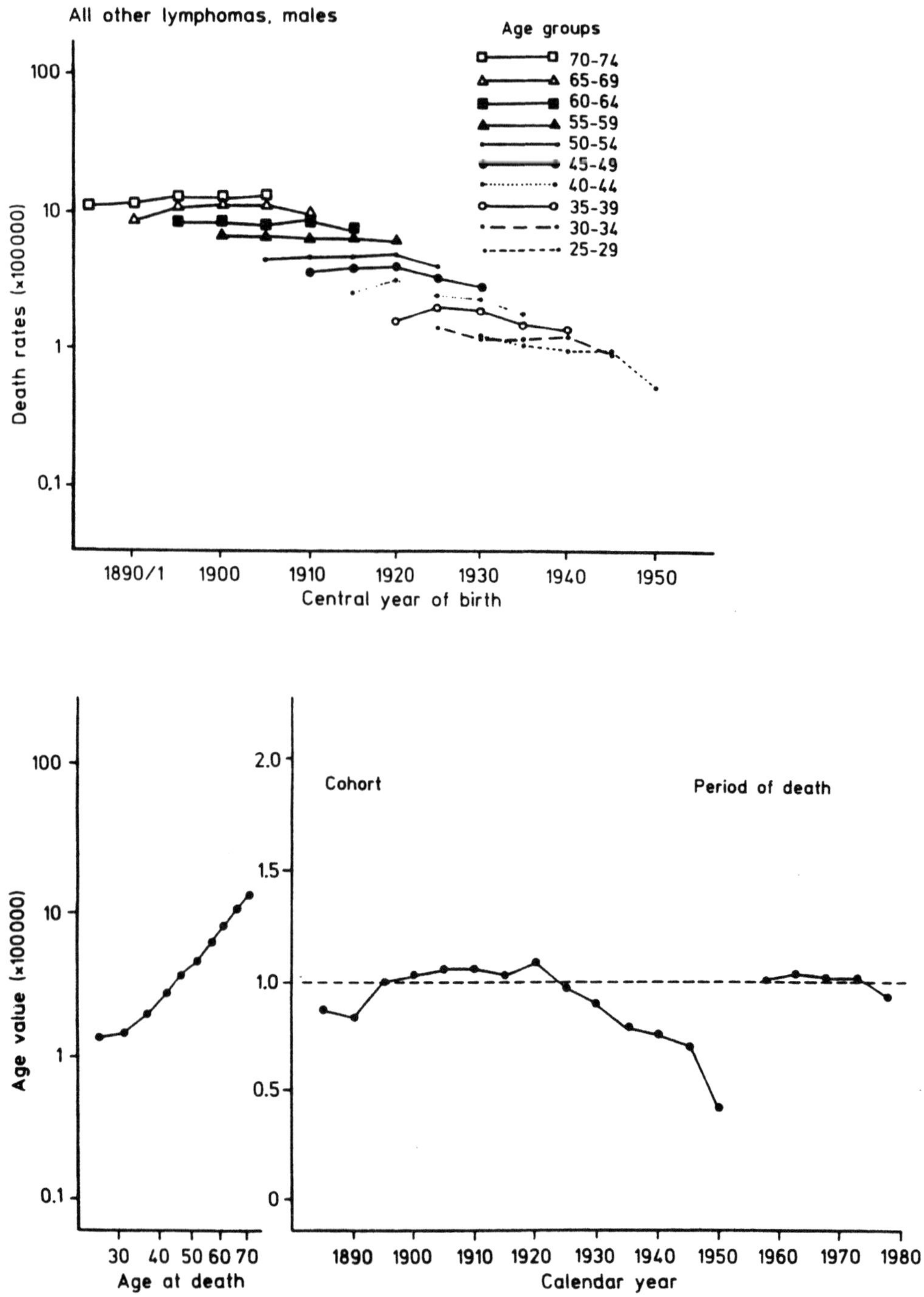

Fig. 3. Mortality from non-Hodgkin's lymphoma by birth cohort in Italy (1955-79) [5]

Temporal Trends

The poor quality of most historical data casts doubts on the interpretation of temporal trends. In the United States the incidence of NHL increased more than 100% from the late 1940s to the early 1980s [8]. These increases are larger than those observed in the mortality rates, which halted in their ascent during the 1970s. Increases in age-adjusted incidence are due primarily to increases of 130% and more among persons aged 65 and over. Increases in mortality rates also were greater in the oldest age groups, each progressively younger group experiencing successively smaller increases. A plateau in mortality rates has occurred in the middle age groups since the late 1960s, and marked decreases have occurred among young people. The pronounced increases in incidence and mortality rates among the older age groups suggest an effect of improved diagnosis among the elderly. Also, part of the overall increases may be attributed to the technological advances of lymphoma classification. Conversely, declines observed in mortality rates among the young are probably due to improvements in the treatment of this cancer [8,9].

Similar increases in NHL mortality have been reported in most European countries, but the declining rates in young people are less clear [9,10]. In England and Wales, cohort curves were increasing up to the 1945 generation, whereas in Italy marked decreases of NHL mortality started earlier, with the 1930 generation [5] (Fig. 3). It is, however, worthwhile remembering that modern treatments are less effective for NHL than for Hodgkin's disease. It is possible, therefore, that the declining U.S. and Italian mortality trends are biased by misclassification of a certain number of Hodgkin's disease cases as NHL.

Socio-Economic and Urban-Rural Gradients

Mortality from NHL shows a positive gradient with socio-economic status and urban residence [9]. A state-by-state survey in the United States revealed elevated mortality rates in coastal California and the Midwest and lower than average rates in the southeast [11,12]. This pattern may reflect socioeconomic factors, particularly social class, urbanisation, and ethnicity, with higher rates seen in countries with many residents of Russian (mainly Jewish) or Greek ancestry [12]. It is noteworthy that the risk of NHL is greater among Israelis of Jewish background than other groups in Israel [12]. Earlier diagnostic improvements may, however, underlie the aforementioned positive associations of social class and urbanisation and NHL risk. In Italy, where a small excess of NHL has been reported in the most industrialised Northern area [13], no rural/urban pattern is evident [14], whereas by far the strongest positive correlations on a regional scale emerge with the number of hospital beds and gross internal product [15]. More recently, a significant excess of NHL cases have been reported in some rural areas [11] and have been associated with various agricultural occupations (see Analytical Epidemiology). A very careful analysis of the distribution of cases of leukaemia and allied disorders occurring in 151 administrative districts from England, Wales and Scotland during 1984 highlighted elevated rates for NHL in rural Yorkshire districts [16]. In view of the uncertainties regarding the accuracy and completeness of NHL diagnoses from cancer registries and other sources over different periods of time, the experience of the Yorkshire Regional Lymphoma Histopathological Panel [17] is worth mentioning. In four district health authorities the ascertainment of lymphoid malignancy cases by

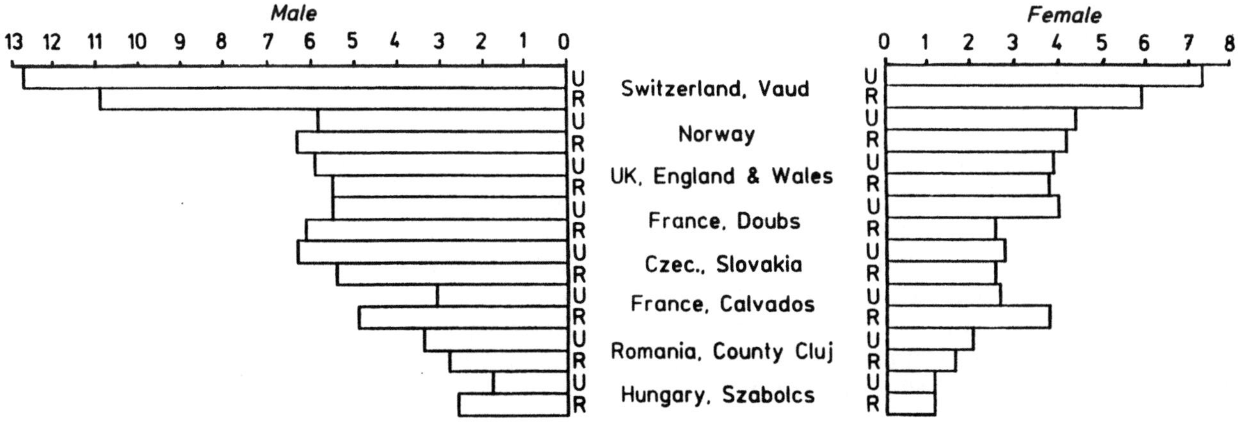

Fig. 4. Average age-standardised incidence rates per 100,000 in urban (U) and rural (R) areas for non-Hodgkin's lymphoma (ICD-9 200-202) in European cancer registries (1978-1982) [6]

the regional cancer registry was contrasted with a specially designed search for records and pathology material which was then submitted to critical review, irrespective of the original diagnosis [10]. Age- and sex-standardised incidence rates for histologically confirmed NHL cases increased from 4,86/100.000 in 1963-67 to 6,86/100.000 in 1978-82 ($p < 0,001$). The greatest increase was displayed by follicular lymphomas, whereas diffuse forms tended to show a relative decrease [10]. Furthermore, it emerged that a large proportion of cancer registry cases were never subjected to histopathological diagnosis (approximately 17%) [10].

Analytical Epidemiology

Severe Immunological Abnormalities

The only well-identified risk factor for NHL is the presence of a severe impairment of the immunological system, either spontaneous or acquired [18,19]. Excesses of NHL, but not of Hodgkin's disease, have been reported in patients affected by rare conditions such as ataxia-teleangectasia, Wiskott-Aldrich syndrome and congenital agammaglobulinaemia [18]. A reliable quantification of the magnitude of the increased risk in spontaneous immunological abnormalities is prevented by various considerations: 1) subjects affected are very few and have a short lifespan; 2) the distinction of true malignant lymphomas from unusual forms of reactivity in immuno-deficient patients with frequent infections is not easy; and 3) over-representation of subjects with rare cancers is likely to occur in immunodeficiency cancer registries, such as that established world-wide in 1973 [20], where there is no detailed information on the patient populations from which cases were drawn.

As regards acquired immunodeficiencies, a several-fold increased risk of NHL has been shown in patients following renal transplantation [21,22]. Lymphoid malignancies start to appear within a few months of the transplant procedure and, interestingly, large-cell lymphomas predominate [22] and there is also an unusual predilection for developing primary lymphoma of the central nervous system. Such a pattern resembles very closely the increase in NHL incidence described in subjects at high-risk of Human Immunodeficiency Virus (HIV) infection, particularly as regards predominance of extranodal, high-grade lymphomas [23-25].

Other Medical Conditions

Although a very strong risk factor, severe immunological impairment is so rare that it accounts for a very small proportion of NHL cases in the general population, in whom the determinants of the malignancy remain largely obscure. Aetiological links with milder aspects of disturbed or aberrant immunity, in addition to genetic factors and infectious agents, were suggested in a very large case-control study in Yorkshire, Great Britain [26,27], which showed significant associations of NHL with past history of skin conditions, malignancies, kidney calculus, pneumonia, scarlet fever and diabetes [27]. Among the conditions affecting the immune system that were assessed in another study conducted in the North-eastern part of Italy on 208 NHL cases and 401 hospital controls, only chronic infectious diseases seemed to confer a significantly elevated risk [28] (Table 1). An increased risk of mortality from lymphosarcoma was suggested in a British cohort of tuberculous patients (Peto J, personal communication). Also Tielchs et al. [29] investigated the relationship between NHL and various acquired disorders potentially affecting the immune system but failed to find an increased risk in patients with a positive history of chronic infectious diseases. Apparent discrepancy may derive from different times of onset of such conditions. In the Italian study [28], all cases of malaria and tuberculosis, reported in excess by NHL patients as compared to control subjects, occurred prior to the 1950s, that is, prior to the availability of effective antibiotic treatment. Such infections may thus have produced, at the time, a truly persistent antigenic stimulus, whereas more recently such diseases may rather have to be considered acute infections.

Table 1. Distribution of 208 cases of non-Hodgkin's lymphoma and 401 hospital controls according to history of various disorders related to the immune system [28]

Disease	Non-Hodgkin's lymphoma No.	(%)	Controls No.	(%)	Relative* risk	95% Confidence interval
Chronic infectious diseases						
None	167	(80)	359	(90)	1	
≥ 1	41	(20)	42	(10)	1.81	(1.13-2.91)
Chronic inflammatory diseases						
None	195	(94)	375	(93)	1	
≥ 1	13	(6)	26	(7)	0.93	(0.47-1.82)
Autoimmune diseases						
None	198	(95)	388	(97)	1	
≥ 1	10	(5)	13	(3)	1.20	(0.52-2.76)
Allergic conditions						
None	164	(79)	315	(79)	1	
≥ 1	44	(21)	86	(21)	0.96	(0.63-1.46)
Herpes zoster						
No	187	(90)	375	(94)	1	
Yes	21	(10)	26	(6)	1.39	(0.74-2.61)
≤ 2 years before diagnosis or interview	4		3			
3-9 years before diagnosis or interview	7		8			
≥ 10 years before diagnosis or interview	10		15			

* Adjusted for age and sex by means of the Mantel-Haenszel procedure [45]

It has been shown that immunosuppression can facilitate episodes of herpes zoster and human papillomavirus infections [30]. In the study by Franceschi et al. [28], a past history of skin warts or condylomata acuminata was not, however, reported more frequently by NHL cases as compared to controls. Conversely, past episodes of herpes zoster infection seemed to be more common among these cases, at least in the ten years preceding the onset of neoplasia. A similar relationship, with the greatest risk near the time of NHL diagnosis, was reported by Cartwright et al. [16]. Paffenberger et al. [31] found that varicella, a childhood infection caused by herpes zoster, was predictive of NHL in adulthood. The excess of episodes of herpes zoster infection may suggest that the persistence of such slow-acting virus may either predispose to development of lymphoma or be favoured by the impairment of the immune system possibly related to the early phases of NHL. It is worth noting that all associations with immune-related diseases found in the Italian investigation [28] emerged most strongly among high-grade NHL, which are those that seem to have been increasing since the spread of HIV [24]. Similarly, in the only other epidemiological study in which an accurate subtype analysis was performed [27], the largest excesses of signs of poor or aberrant immunity (e.g. steroid and antihistamine use, eczema, herpes simplex infections, etc.) were found in high-grade lymphomas [27].

Occupation

In the occupational field, employment in agriculture and forestry [32-34] and, in particular, exposure to phenoxy acid, chlorophenols and organic solvents [35] and insecticides [32], have been suggested as causative factors in NHL, but other studies failed to confirm the association, at least with the significance originally suggested [36]. Increased risks have also been suspected among workers exposed to wood [27,37], epoxy glues [27], food [12] and meat [34]. In the aforementioned Italian case-control study [28], there was a hint that employment in chemical and petrochemical industries may increase the probability of the onset of NHL, in agreement with a few previous reports (Table 2) [38,39]. The elevation of risk, however, did not tend to be higher in those individuals who had been employed in such industries for longer periods.

Diet

The only published case-control study in which information on diet was elicited was conducted in Italy [40]. Some dietary habits turned out to affect NHL risk, including high intake of milk, liver, fats in seasoning and methylxanthine-containing beverages.
Conversely, relatively high consumption of whole-grain bread and pasta seemed to act protectively (Table 3). On an international scale, strong positive correlations emerged between NHL and dairy products (correlation coefficient r=0.70), and all animal proteins (r=0.67), whereas vegetal foods exibited non-significant negative coefficients [41]. In analogy with experimental data, where augmentation of dietary proteins, namely casein, increased the number of lymphomas in rats [42], such geographical correlations were mainly interpreted as evidence that excessive

Table 2. Relative risk of Non-Hodgkin's lymphoma according to selected ocupations and exposures * [28]

Occupation or exposure	Non-Hodgkin's lymphoma No. of exposed	Controls No. of exposed	Relative# risk	95% Confidence interval
Chemical workers	20	27	1.64	(0.88-3.06)
Petrochemical workers	15	18	1.83	(0.87-3.84)
Dye and paint	14	38	0.72	(0.36-1.44)
Plastic resin and glue	10	21	1.01	(0.46-2.23)
Benzene and solvents	15	28	1.14	(0.57-2.28)
Wood and furniture workers	18	55	0.66	(0.37-1.19)
Metal and metal dust	19	37	1.10	(0.61-1.99)
Meat workers	26	36	1.11	(0.64-1.90)
Herbicides and pesticides	22	35	1.01	(0.58-1.77)

* Only occupations and exposures which involved at least ten cases
# Adjusted for age and sex by means of the Mantel-Haenszel procedure [45,46]

Table 3. Foods or groups of foods significantly related to non-Hodgkin's lymphoma risk [40]

Food item	Model	Relative risk estimates [a] for level of consumption			X^2_1 (trend)
		Low	Intermediate	High	
Whole-grain bread or pasta	A [a]	1	0.77	0.45	6.59 [c]
	B [b]	1	0.80	0.44	6.41 [c]
Liver	A [a]	1	1.38	1.69	3.99 [d]
	B [b]	1	1.30	1.63	3.12
Milk	A [a]	1	1.37	2.37	10.45 [c]
	B [b]	1	1.31	2.17	7.96 [c]
Fats in seasoning	A [a]	1	1.33	2.04	9.42 [c]
	B [b]	1	1.31	1.75	5.50 [d]
Methylxantine-containing beverages	A [a]	1	1.29	1.77	4.58 [d]
	B [b]	1	1.26	1.69	3.63

a Model including terms for age, sex, education, weight and smoking status [47]
b Model including the same non-dietary variables plus all the above-listed food items
c $p < 0.01$
d $p < 0.05$

absorption of food proteins and fats, only partly blocked by the gastro-intestinal mucous membrane, induces harmful chronic hyper-stimulation of the immune system [41]. Lymphomas are, in fact, one-hundred times more common in individuals with coeliac disease than in the general population [43].
High dietary fibre intake has been shown to decrease the risk of some cancers (e.g. colon cancer) in populations consuming diets high in fat and proteins [42]. Since fat and/or animal proteins seem to be positively correlated to risk of NHL in the present data set, it can be hypothesised that alimentary fibres may affect dilution, absorption or breakdown of such compounds in the gut, either directly or by modifying the gut microflora composition.

Conclusion

The difficulties of studying the epidemiology of NHL have been stressed repeatedly in the present review. Analyses of geographical and temporal trends are hampered by classification difficulties, whereas relatively few case-control studies have been conducted on this subject.
Apart from severe abnormalities of the immunological system, no strong association with NHL has emerged, in spite of the large number of potential risk factors investigated in the case-control studies [27-29,40]. Other analytic epidemiological studies should be encouraged and directed towards the few clues deriving from previous observations,

namely the increasing incidence of NHL, particularly of bad-prognosis, high-grade, extranodal types, the potential role of viral infections, occupational and environmental exposures and dietary habits. It would be also particularly fruitful to develop ways to distinguish different types of NHL and, possibly, to assess milder signs of impairments of the immunological status sufficiently simple to be applied to large-scale epidemiological research.

Acknowledgements

The author thanks Dr. Renato Talamini, Dr. Ettore Bidoli, Ilaria Calderan and Anna Redivo for technical assistance. This work was supported by the Italian League against Tumours and the Italian Association for Cancer Research.

REFERENCES

1 Magrath IT: Lymphocyte differentiation: An essential basis for the comprehension of lymphoid neoplasia. JNCI 1981 (67):501-514
2 National Cancer Institute sponsored study of classifications of non-Hodgkin's lymphoma. Summary and description of a working formulation for clinical usage. The non-Hodgkin's lymphoma pathologic classification project. Cancer 1982 (49):2112-2135
3 Ultmann JE, Jacobs RH: The non-Hodgkin's lymphomas. Cancer 1985 (35):66-85
4 WHO International Classification of Diseases. Manual of the international statistical classification of diseases, injuries and causes of death. Based on the recommendations of the Ninth Revision Conference 1975 and adopted by the 29th World Health Assembly. World Health Assembly. World Health Organization, Geneva 1977
5 Decarli A, La Vecchia C, Cislaghi C, Fasoli M, Mezzanotte G, Negri E: La mortalità per tumori in Italia, 1955-1979: Effetti dell'età, della generazione di nascita e del periodo di morte. Monografie L.I.C.T. 1986 (4):1-72
6 Muir C, Waterhouse J, Mack T, Powell J, Whelan S: Cancer Incidence in Five Continents. Volume V. IARC Scientific Publication no. 88. International Agency for Research on Cancer, Lyon 1987
7 Waterhouse J, Muir C, Correa P, Powell J: Cancer Incidence in Five Continents. Volume III. IARC Scientific Publication no. 15. International Agency for Research on Cancer, Lyon 1976
8 Devesa SS, Silverman DT, Young JL Jr, Pollack ES, Brown CC, Horm JW, Percy CL, Myers MH, McKay FW, Fraumeni JF Jr: Cancer incidence and mortality trends among whites in the United States, 1947-84. JNCI 1987 (79):701-770
9 Greene MH: Non-Hodgkin's lymphoma and mycosis fungoides. In: Schottenfeld D, Fraumeni JF Jr (eds) Cancer Epidemiology and Prevention. Saunders, Philadelphia 1982. pp 754-778
10 Barnes N, Cartwright RA, O'Brien CO, Richards IDG, Roberts B, Bird CC: Rising incidence of lymphoid malignancies - True or false? Br J Cancer 1986 (53):393-398
11 Pickle LW, Mason TJ, Howard N, Hoover R, Fraumeni JF Jr: Atlas of U.S. cancer mortality among whites:1950-1980. U.S. Department of Health and Human Services, DHHS Publication No (NIH) 87-2900. Washington 1987
12 Cantor KR, Fraumeni FJ Jr: Distribution of non-Hodgkin's lymphoma in the United States between 1950 and 1975. Cancer Res 1980 (40):2645-2652
13 Mezzanotte G, Cislaghi C, Decarli A, La Vecchia C: Cancer mortality in broad Italian geographical areas, 1975-77. Tumori 1986 (72):145-152
14 Cislaghi C, Decarli A, La Vecchia C, Laverda N, Mezzanotte G, Smans M: Dati indicatori e mappe di mortalità tumorale. Italia 1975-1977. Pitagora, Bologna 1986
15 Decarli A, La Vecchia C: Environmental factors and cancer mortality in Italy: Correlation exercise. Oncology 1986 (43):116-126
16 Barnes N, Beddal AC, Bird CC, Bradfield JWB, Brown IL, Burnett AK, Cartwright RA, Davies JD, Edwards MS, Ellis IO, Gillis CR, Goepel JR, Gorst D, Gough J, Hutchinson RM, Al-Ismail SAD, Jones PAE, Lauder I, Lee FD, Lucie NP, Miller JG, Nicholson C, Prentice AG, Richards IDG, Roberts B, Rowe RCG, Southgate J, Turner DR, Whittaker JA, Winfield DA, Wood JK: Distribution of leukemia, lymphoma, and allied diseases in parts of Great Britain: Analysis by administrative districts and simulations of adjacencies. Leukemia 1987 (1):78-81
17 Bird CC, Lauder I, Kellett HS, Chorlton I, Barnes N, Darwin C, Cartwright RA, Boyko R: Yorkshire regional lymphoma histopathology panel: Analysis of five years' experience. J Pathol 1984 (143):249-258
18 UICC International Union Against Cancer: Malignant lymphoma. A series of Workshops on the Biology of Human Cancer Report no. 7. UICC Technical Report Series Vol 37. Geneva 1978
19 Gatti RA, Good RA: Occurrence of malignancy in immunodeficiency diseases. A literature review. Cancer 1971 (28):89-98
20 Filopovich AH: The immunodeficiency cancer registry is renewed. Immunology Today 1984 (5):309
21 Kinlen LJ, Scheil AGR, Peto J, Doll R: Collaborative United Kingdom-Australian study of cancer in patients treated with immunosuppressive drugs. Br Med J 1979 (2):1461-1466
22 Hoover R: Effects of Drugs-Immunosuppression. In: Origins of Human Cancer. Cold Spring Harbor laboratory no. 7, New York 1977
23 Ross R, Dworsky R, Paganini-Hill A, Levine A, Mack T: Non-Hodgkin's lymphomas in never-married men in Los Angeles. Br J Cancer 1985 (52):785-787
24 Chase Boring C, Brynes RK, Chan WC, Causey N, Gregory HR, Nadel MR, Greenberg R: Increase in high-grade lymphomas in young men. Lancet 1985 (i):857-859

25 Biggar RJ, Horm J, Goedert J, Melbye M: Cancer in a group at risk of acquired immunodeficiency syndrome (AIDS) through 1984. Am J Epidemiol 1987 (126):578-586
26 Bernard SM, Cartwright RA, Bird CC, Gerald Richards ID, Lauder I, Roberts BE: Aetiologic factors in lymphoid malignancies: a case-control epidemiological study. Leuk Res 1984 (8):681-689
27 Cartwright RA, McKinney PA, O'Brien C, Richards IDG, Roberts B, Lauder I, Darwin CM, Bernard SM, Bird CC: Non-Hodgkin's lymphoma: case control epidemiological study in Yorkshire. Leuk Res 1988 (12):81-88
28 Franceschi S, Serraino D, Bidoli E, Talamini R, Tirelli U, Carbone A, La Vecchia C: The epidemiology on Non-Hodgkin's lymphoma in the North-East of Italy: a hospital-based case-control study. Leuk Res 1989 (in press)
29 Tielsch JM, Linet MS, Szklo M: Acquired disorders affecting the immune system and non-Hodgkin's lymphoma. Prev Med 1987 (16):96-106
30 Boyle J, MacKie RM, Briggs JD, Junor BFR: Cancer, warts, and sunshine in renal transplant patients. Lancet 1984 (i):702-705
31 Paffenbarger RSJr, Wing AL, Hyde RT: Characteristics in youth predictive of adult-onset malignant lymphomas, melanomas, and leukemias: Brief communication. JNCI 1978 (60): 89-92
32 Cantor KP: Farming and mortality from non-Hodgkin's lymphoma: A case-control study. Int J Cancer 1982 (29):239-247
33 Pearce NE, Smith AH, Fischer DO: Malignant lymphoma and multiple myeloma linked with agricultural occupations in a New Zealand cancer registry-based study. Am J Epidemiol 1985 (121):225-237
34 Pearce NE, Sheppard RA, Smith AH, Teague CA: Non-Hodgkin's lymphoma and farming: An expanded case-control study. Int J Cancer 1987 (39):155-161
35 Hardell L, Eriksson M, Lenner P, Lundgren E: Malignant lymphoma and exposure to chemicals, especially organic solvents, chlorophenols and phenoxy acids: A case-control study. Br J Cancer 1981 (43):169-17
36 Wiklund K, Dich J, Holm LE: Risk of malignant lymphoma in Swedish pesticide appliers. Br J Cancer 1987 (56):505-508
37 Grufferman S, Duong T, Cole P: Occupation and Hodgkin's disease. JNCI 1976 (57):1193-1195
38 Li FP, Fraumeni JF, Mantel N, Miller RW: Cancer mortality among chemists. JNCI 1969 (43):1159-1164
39 Olin R: Leukaemia and Hodgkin's disease among Swedish chemistry graduates. Lancet 1976 (ii):916
40 Franceschi S, Serraino D, Carbone A, Talamini R, La Veccia C: Dietary factors and Non-Hodgkin's lymphoma: A case-control study in the North-eastern part of Italy. Nutr Cancer 1989 (in press)
41 Cunningham AS: Lymphomas and animal-protein consumption. Lancet 1976 (ii):1184-1186
42 Ross MH, Bras GJ: Tumor incidence patterns and nutrition in the rat. J Nutr 1965 (87):245-260
43 Harris OD, Cooke WT, Thompson H, Waterhouse JAH: Malignancy in adult coeliac disease and idiopathic steatorrhoea. Am J Med 1967 (42):899-912
44 Reddy BS: Dietary fiber and colon cancer: Animal model studies. Prev Med 1987 (16):559-565
45 Mantel N, Haenszel W: Statistical aspects of the analysis of data from retrospective studies of disease. JNCI 1959 (22):719-748
46 Mantel N: Chi-square tests with one degree of freedom: Extension of the Mantel-Haenszel procedure. J Am Stat Assoc 1963 (58):690-700
47 Breslow NE, Day NE: Statistical Methods in Cancer Research: The Analysis of Case-Control studies. IARC Scientific Publication 32, Lyon 1980. pp 192-246

Pathological Classification of Non-Hodgkin's Lymphomas in Europe

Paul-André Bryon and Francoise Berger

Haematopathology and Analytical Cytology Laboratory, Université Claude-Bernard, Faculté de Médecine Lyon-Nord, Domaine Rockefeller, 69373 Lyon, France

In recent years, European haematopathologists have contributed enormously to the improvement of non-Hodgkin's lymphomas (NHL) classification. Through the European Lymphoma Club, EORTC trials and other co-operative studies, they have helped to refine diagnostic criteria and to improve current classifications. The recent creation of the "European Association for Haematopathology" is a result of the European scientific productiveness in this field. The present paper is only a summary of the current state of NHL classification. Although it is intended as an outline of the current status of NHL classification in Europe, it will also mention some significant results from North-America and Japan.

Recently Described or Refined Entities

A greater precision in cytohistological identification and a wider use of the immunological characterisation of NHL has led to a better definition of many lymphomas of B-cell and T-cell origin and to a refinement of their classification. New clinicopathologic entities are emerging as distinctive diseases with their own prognostic significance.

Lymphomas of the Mucosa-Associated Lymphoid Tissue: MALT

Isaacson and Wright have suggested that many extranodal lymphomas, particularly those of the gastrointestinal tract, lung, salivary gland and thyroid, could arise from mucosa-associated lymphoid tissue (MALT) [1]. Tumoural cells have a tendency to invade epithelial structures, giving rise to lympho-epithelial lesions, and to infiltrate pre-existing reactive lymphoid follicles, frequently producing a pseudo-follicular appearance [2,3]. This pattern, together with the presence of the reactive lymphoid follicles and the generally good prognosis, explained why some of these tumours were originally described as "pseudo-lymphoma". Immunohistochemistry and gene-rearrangement studies have shown these tumours to be clonal in origin. Current histological classifications of nodal NHL are difficult to apply to these tumours.
The commonest form is characterised by the presence of small "centrocyte-like" cells within a mixed population of small lymphocytes, lymphoplasmacytoid cells and plasma cells giving sometimes an "immunocytoma-like" appearance. Occasionally, a single cell type predominates. The centrocyte-like cells probably arise from a special type of extra-follicular (parafollicular) small cells bearing close similarities to marginal zone cells which were defined as a distinct non-circulating B-cell lineage [4]. Large blastic cells, morphologically similar to centroblasts and immunoblasts, are found in variable proportion, and they are sometimes predominant. However, in some instances, these large-cell lymphomas appear to be arising from a small-cell lymphoma with the presence of small cells and lymphoepithelial lesions in adjacent sections.
According to Isaacson, the overall prognosis of this form of MALT tumour is considerably better than that of nodal tumours of similar

histological grade. These tumours tend to remain localised until late in the course of the disease and hence often respond favourably to local therapy. But the term "MALT lymphoma" is imprecise and does not necessarily imply a good prognosis. Some observations suggest that this lymphoma represents a spectrum of morphological forms and that transition from low to high grade may occur. According to Hall et al., such tumours may be assigned to high grade if the large cell component is greater than 20% [5].
Multiple lymphomatous polyposis is a distinctive entity defined by multifocal lesions. The polyps may affect the whole gut or be centred in one area. This tumour is composed of centrocytes (small cleaved and/or intermediate lymphocytic). This disease is more aggressive than the other low-grade lymphomas of the MALT [5].

Enteropathy-Associated T-cell Lymphoma

This lymphoma, originally described as "malignant histiocytosis of the intestine", complicates coeliac disease and appears to arise from a variety of T-lymphocytes homing in the gut mucosa [6]. Multiple tumour localisations may be found within the intestine with little evidence of dissemination elsewhere. Adjacent intestine may show an intense infiltration of the mucosal epithelium with T-lymphocytes, as in severe coeliac disease. Other peripheral T-cell lymphomas of the gastrointestinal tract without associated coeliac disease have been described and they have a bad prognosis [7].

Monocytoid B-cell Lymphoma

The term "monocytoid B-cell lymphoma" (MBCL) [8] has been proposed for a new B-cell neoplasm characterised by cells exhibiting the same morphological and immunological features as reactive "monocytoid B-cells" previously described in reactive lymphadenopathies [9,10]. Monocytoid B lymphocytes have also been reported as one neoplastic component in some low-grade lymphomas including small lymphocytic and small cleaved types. Therefore, the pure MBCL may be confused with other diffuse small B-cell lymphoproliferative disorders, particularly hairy cell leukaemia (HCL). There are remarkable morphologic and phenotypic similarities between MBCL and HCL. But patients with MBCL rarely have bone marrow involvement, significant splenomegaly, leukaemic conversion and pancytopenia whereas patients with HCL only rarely have lymph-node involvement. In the past, because of a lack of well-defined criteria, MBCL has been confused with the other lymphoproliferative disorders. MBCL has the same age distribution as the other low-grade lymphomas. Similar to other low-grade lymphomas, MBCL may progress to a higher grade lymphoma of large blastic cell type.

Large Cell Anaplastic (Ki-1) Positive Lymphoma

This entity has been recognised using the monoclonal antibody Ki-1 assigned to CD 30 [11]. This antibody, like the more recently available Ber-H2 antibody, recognises an activation antigen present on activated T and B lymphocytes. These antibodies react with the Sternberg-Reed cells and Hodgkin's cells of Hodgkin's disease, but also with some cells of non-Hodgkin's T-cell and, less commonly, B-cell lymphomas. Thus, the diagnosis of Ki-1 lymphoma must be restricted to the type of lymphoma in which every neoplastic cell stains strongly with the Ki-1 (or Ber-H2) antibody. This tumour may frequently express epithelial membrane antigen (EMA) but it is negative for cytokeratin. About one third of the cases lack the leukocyte common antigen. This lymphoma is mainly composed of very large neoplastic cells with abundant pale or moderately basophilic cytoplasm (grey in Giemsa staining) and large irregular nuclei. Some cells may resemble Sternberg-Reed cells. Most of the cells of these tumours are frequently positive for both anti-Tac (Il-2 receptor) and HLA class II antigen. These tumours express T-cell, less frequently B-cell or, in very rare instances, monocytic antigens. The immunophenotype of the T-cell tumour is often incomplete, and lineage specific markers may be totally absent (null type).
The tendency of the neoplastic cells to form seemingly cohesive pseudo-metastatic

sheets has sometimes led to the misdiagnosis of anaplastic carcinoma. The frequent sinusoidal permeation, together with the common accompaniment of large actively phagocytic macrophages, gave rise to the term "malignant histiocytosis" frequently used for these tumours in the past. The term "large cell anaplastic lymphoma" has been proposed for this type [12]. According to age, two groups can be identified: the younger group (<20 years) has a relatively better prognosis than the older group. But the use of intensive chemotherapeutic protocols improves the prognosis of this tumour [13]. Ki-1 positive large-cell anaplastic lymphomas may appear in some cases to be "secondary", occurring after low-grade non-Hodgkin lymphomas as well as after Hodgkin's lymphomas.

Mediastinal B Large-cell Lymphoma

B-cell lymphoma of the thymus is a clinicopathological entity that has only recently been recognised. Many cases were, in the past, erroneously diagnosed as Hodgkin's disease, T-cell lymphoma, and even thymic carcinoma. The distinctive clinical feature of this lymphoma is its frequency of occurrence in young adult females. Histologically, this tumour is composed of large cells, with a diffuse growth pattern, frequently with pleomorphic nuclei and sometimes clear cytoplasms [14]. Multinucleated cells resembling Reed-Sternberg cells may be present. Bands of sclerosis are frequent [15] and this can lead to confusion with thymic carcinoma. The features of this type of lymphoma do not fit easily into any of the current classifications of NHL. According to Isaacson, this lymphoma is derived from a thymic resident population of B-cells [16]. It appears clinically of high grade, best treated with aggressive chemotherapy [17].

Angiocentric Immunoblastic Lymphoma and Lethal Midline Granuloma

These entities, probably heterogeneous, include some T-cell nasopharyngeal lymphomas and angiocentric immunoproliferative lymphomas such as Liebow's lymphomatoid granulomatosis [18,19]. Besides the histologic lesions of pleomorphic peripheral T-cell NHL, these diseases may show a special lesion of vessels with predominant vessel involvement. Although locally destructive, they may remain localised for long periods of time, with death resulting from local infiltration.

Update of Current Non-Hodgkin's Lymphoma Classifications

Two classification systems are mainly used in Europe: the Kiel Classification (KC) and the Working Formulation (WF). The advantages and the limitations of these two systems are well known and they have been widely discussed [20-22]. The KC, based on physiopathological and immunological criteria, is used by the majority of European pathologists in preference to other systems. The Working Formulation, a compromise between the Rappaport and Lukes-Collins classifications, is often required in Europe for clinical studies and cooperative trials.
The KC has been updated recently by the members of the European Lymphoma Club, with some refinements and a clearer distinction between B-cell and T-cell NHL (Table 1) [23]. Some improvements of the WF have also been suggested in recent years [22-25]. It seems necessary to include in the WF some of the new entities that are well accepted at the moment in Europe, and to distinguish between B- and T-NHL (Table 2). Thus, all the main entities may be defined in these two classification systems, but the translation from one system into another is difficult for some subtypes without true equivalence between the two classifications: for instance, centroblastic polymorphous, centrocytic diffuse, lymphoplasmacytic polymorphic etc.

B-cell Lymphomas

Follicular lymphomas are recognised on the basis of their nodular pattern. It is now well established that they are derived from follicle centre cells and composed of cells that morphologically resemble the normal centrocytes (small-cleaved cells) and cen-

Table 1. Updated Kiel classification of Non-Hodgkin's Lymphomas

B-cell	T-cell
Low grade	**Low grade**
*Lymphocytic-chronic lymphocytic and hairy cell leukaemia	Lymphocytic-chronic lymphocytic and prolymphocytic leukaemia
	Small, cerebriform cell-mycosis fungoides, Sezary's syndrome
Lymphoplasmacytic/cytoid	Lymphoepithelial (Lennert's)
Plasmacytic	Angioimmunoblastic (AILD, Lg X)
*Centroblastic/centrocytic	
-follicular ± diffuse	T-zone
-diffuse	Pleomorphic, small cell
Centrocytic	(HTLV-1±)
High grade	**High grade**
Centroblastic	Pleomorphic, medium and large cell (HTLV-1±)
*Immunoblastic	Immunoblastic (HTLV-1±)
*Large cell anaplastic (Ki-1)	Large cell anaplastic (Ki-1)
Burkitt's lymphoma	
*Lymphoblastic	Lymphoblastic
Rare types	**Rare types**

*Indicates some degree of correspondence, either in morphology, or in functional expression, between categories in two columns

troblasts (large non-cleaved cells) of reactive follicles. These lymphomas may have a follicular, or a follicular and diffuse growth pattern. Recognition of the follicular pattern is a basic feature of the WF, whereas the KC is mainly based on the recognition of the cytologic type, with the designation of the follicular and/or diffuse pattern as an additional feature. The proportion of small and large cells in follicular lymphomas varies. The most frequent type consists predominantly of centrocytes and is designated as **follicular predominantly small-cleaved** in the WF and **centroblastic-centrocytic**, follicular, small cell, in the KC. The proportion of large cells is higher in other types, for instance greater than 30% in the **follicular mixed** of the WF, and greater than 50% in the **follicular large cell** of the WF, corresponding to the **centroblastic** type, follicular, of the KC. Precise criteria for the subdivision of follicular lymphomas need to be established. Thus, the subdivision according to the cell size and morphology is difficult, probably not very reproducible, and could benefit from more objective methods than the conventional histologic analysis. Disease progression usually results in increased numbers of large (centroblastic) cells and progressive loss of the follicular pattern.

Diffuse small B-cell lymphomas may theoretically be grouped into two main types: 1) diffuse small non-centrofollicular cells mainly represented by lymphocytic (or prolymphocytic) and lymphoplasmacytic/cytoid lymphomas, and 2) diffuse small follicle centre cells corresponding to the diffuse pattern counterpart of follicular lymphomas.

Small lymphocytic lymphoma is defined by a monotonous proliferation of small, round lymphocytes with clumped chromatin structure. The pattern is diffuse, but pseudofollicular "growth centres" may be seen. When cells with proeminent central nucleoli are predominant, the tumour is termed as "prolymphocytic". A plasma cell differentiation defined the lymphoplasmacytic type.

Table 2. A classification scheme of the Working Formulation, modified for including some subcategories used in European clinical studies and expanded for peripheral T-cell malignant lymphomas

WF (main category)	B-cell subcategory	T-cell subcategory
A. Small lymphocytic	Lymphocytic (B)	Lymphocytic (T)
	Lympho-plasmocytoid	
	Prolymphocytic (B)	Prolymphocytic (T)
B. Follicular small-cleaved	Follicular	
	Diffuse areas	
C. Follicular mixed	Follicular	
	Diffuse areas	
D. Follicular large	Large cleaved	
	Large non-cleaved	
	Multilobated	
	Diffuse areas	
E. Diffuse small/medium	Intermediate lymphocytic	
	Mantle-zone	T-zone
	Small-cleaved	Small pleomorphous
F. Diffuse mixed	Follicular centre cells	Lymphoepithelioid
	Lympho-plasmacytic polymorphous	Angioimmunoblastic-like
G. Diffuse large	Cleaved	
	Non-cleaved	
	Multi-lobated	
	Polymorphous	
H. Immunoblastic	Monomorphous (B)	Immunoblastic (T)
	Polymorphous (B)	Polymorphous (T)
		Clear/pale cells
I. Lymphoblastic	Lymphoblastic (B)	Lymphoblastic (T)
		Convoluted/non-convoluted
J. Small non-cleaved Burkitt's	Monomorphous	
	Polymorphous non-Burkitt's	
Miscellaneous		
K.		Mycosis fungoides
L.	Extramedullary plasmocytoma	
M.	Large-cell anaplastic	Ki-1 +
N. Composite		
O. Unclassifiable/Other		

Diffuse small cleaved and diffuse mixed lymphomas are defined as the diffuse pattern counterpart of follicular lymphomas.

The sub-classification of small B-cell lymphomas may be difficult for three main reasons: 1) The cell composition is often heterogeneous with a mixed population of small lymphocytes, small-cleaved cells (centrocytes), lymphoplasmacytoid cells and larger cells in varying proportions. 2) The recognition of the plasmacytic/cytoid differentiation, which is the basic criterion of the immunocytoma of the KC, is an accessory feature in the WF, so that immunocytoma may correspond to subtypes A or F of the WF, presenting problems for interpreting the prognostic significance of this entity. 3) In the KC, "centrocytic" lymphoma is interpreted as distinct from diffuse follicle centre cell lymphomas and as arising from a non-centrofollicular cell in an extrafollicular site (mantle zone: in the earliest form of this disease, the tumour cells from the mantle zone diffusely infiltrate the lymph node, producing a "mantle zone" pattern). Thus, it is unfortunate that in the KC the same term "centrocyte" has been used to designate 1) the small cleaved cell of the follicular centroblastic/centrocytic lymphomas and 2) the cell of diffuse lymphoma equivalent to the tumour designated as "diffuse intermediate cell lymphoma" (and "mantle-zone lymphoma") in the American literature [26,27]. On the other hand, it is unfortunate that this latter entity has not been provided for in the WF.

Large B-cell lymphomas. Among the large B-cell lymphomas, two types are well accepted and now largely used in Europe: centroblastic (large non-cleaved of the WF) and B-immunoblastic. The term "centroblastic" is the more convenient term for defining the group of large centrofollicular cell lymphomas. A clearcut distinction between centroblastic and immunoblastic is often difficult, particularly when the cell population is a mixture of centroblasts and immunoblasts with a large number of transition forms. Centroblastic and immunoblastic lymphomas may arise *ex novo* without any previous history of lymphoma, or secondarily in patients with a previous low-grade lymphoma, follicular for secondary centroblastic lymphoma, lymphocytic or lymphoplasmacytic for secondary immunoblastic lymphoma. Some subtypes of large B-cells are currently used in Europe:

- **large cleaved** of the WF corresponding to the **centroblastic-centrocytoid** subtype described by Lennert [28]
- **large non-cleaved** corresponding to the **centroblastic monomorphic** of the Kiel group [28]
- **centroblastic multilobated**, although initially described as a T-cell lymphoma , now shown to be a well-recognised B-cell entity [29]
- **centroblastic polymorphic** defined by an admixture of centroblasts and immunoblasts with a large number of transition forms. Multilobated and irregular nuclei are sometimes possible, giving the tumour a pleomorphic appearance resembling in some aspects peripheral T-cell lymphomas. According to Lennert, the percentage of immunoblasts in this type could be high, and the diagnosis must be based on the following criterion: "No matter how high the content of immunoblasts, if germinal centre cells are an obvious component" [28]. Such cases would be frequently classified as "immunoblastic" according to the WF, and particularly as "polymorphic B-cell immunoblastic" according to some modified schemes of the WF [25].

B-Immunoblastic is consequently reserved, in the KC, to cases in which immunoblasts (defined by their nuclei with a proeminent central nucleolus) are largely predominant, with less than 10% germinal centre cells. This type is broader according to the WF. Lennert's group has subdivided B-Immunoblastic lymphomas into three subtypes: without plasmacytic differentiation, with plasmacytic differentiation, with rich infiltration of small lymphocytes [28]. This third variant, with a sigificant content of lymphocytes, is interpreted as a secondary immunoblastic lymphoma, occurring secondary to chronic lymphocytic leukaemia or immunocytoma. This variant is the same as "immunoblastic, CLL in Richter's transformation" of a modified WF scheme [25].

Burkitt's lymphoma is characterised by the proliferation of medium-sized basophilic cells often interspersed with histiocytes (starry-sky pattern). This lymphoma is called **small non-cleaved** in the WF. But the tumoral cells may show great variations in cell size and in nucleus morphology. Different morphological variants have been described. Cytological study of European cases and cell lines collected from different countries have confirmed great variations in cell morphology [30,31]. Although the boundaries between the different morphologic variants of Burkitt's lymphoma are not sharp, two main subtypes have been described:

- **Burkitt's type**, defined by the classical criteria proposed at the Bethesda conference, and called "without plasmablastic differentiation" by Lennert's group [28]
- **Small non-cleaved, non-Burkitt's type**, with cellular heterogeneity, variations in the nuclear size, presence of proeminent nucleoli, interpreted as "Burkitt's lymphoma with plasmablastic differentiation" by Lennert [28];

In fact, these two subtypes express the same entity, with the same cytogenetic features. However, the distinction of different morphologic variants could be of interest, to be shown in future studies.

B-Lymphoblastic lymphoma is morphologically indistinguishable from lymphoblastic lymphoma of the T-cell phenotype.

T-cell Lymphomas

T-cell lymphoblastic lymphoma is a well-known entity, closely related to acute lymphoblastic leukaemia. The cases may be classified as "convoluted" or "nonconvoluted" depending on small variations of the nuclear morphology, without immunological or clinical significance.

Peripheral T-cell Lymphomas

The term "peripheral" T-cell lymphoma (PTCL) as been applied to a heterogeneous group of malignant lymphomas other than lymphoblastic, and indicates a post-thymic differentiation. PTCL may appear originally in the skin (epidermotropic PTCL), or in other tissues (non-cutaneous PTCL).

Epidermotropic PTCL. Two clinically distinct dermatopathic entities, Mycosis fungoides and Sezary's Syndrome, initially manifest in the skin and usually show epidermotropism in their early phase, often with Pautrier's pseudo abcesses. Small cells exhibiting extreme nuclear convolutions (hyperconvoluted or cerebriform nuclei) are intermingled with larger atypical cells, especially in cases of mycosis fungoides. In later stages, increasing anaplasia of the cells may result in their transformation into high-grade NHL of pleomorphic type.

Nonepidermotropic PTCL. PTCLs other than epidermotropic NHL have become more easily recognisable in the last decade as a result of the wider use of immunochemistry and in some instances of gene rearrangement studies. They appear to constitute between 10 and 15% of NHL seen in Europe. As a group they are still poorly defined and exhibit marked morphological, immunological and clinical diversity [32]. This heterogeneity makes their classification difficult.

Morphologically, PTCLs exhibit a number of morphological features that may suggest their immunological lineage. Some striking features are: presence of a large number of histiocytes, variable number of eosinophils, presence of high-endothelial postcapillary venules. They frequently involve primarily the T-dependent areas of lymph nodes and spleen, often surrounding isolated reactive germinal follicles. The tumour cells may have a very complex nucleus and may exhibit a clear cytoplasm. None of these features, however, are reliable. An abnormal phenotype (loss of one or more pan-T differentiation antigens) may sometimes be seen. The monoclonality had to be proved by gene rearrangement studies. The presence of large numbers of histiocytes, eosinophils and other reactive cells in some cases of T-cell lymphoma makes it difficult to differentiate between these cases and Hodgkin's disease. Multinucleated cells, showing some resemblance to Reed-Sternberg cells, may occur. Immuno-histochemistry and gene rearrangement studies do not always clarify the differential diagnosis between PTCL and Hodgkin's disease.

Immunophenotypic studies do not provide a valuable means of subclassifying T-cell lymphomas. Investigators in Japan who have had extensive experience with adult PTCLs have subdivided them morphologically into several subtypes. Some of them are now well accepted in Europe [12]. However, this classification still appears to have little clinical backing. Furthermore, in many patients the morphology of PTCL frequently changes with disease progression and even at different sites in the same patient, increasing the difficulty of a precise morphological classification. Nevertheless, morphology provides today a rough means of dividing T-cell lymphomas: some subtypes now currently used are indicated as follows:

Small and Medium-Sized Cell Types

T-zone lymphoma. This term was originally given to a tumour growing in the T-zones and preserving the follicles, which may even be hyperplastic in the early stage of tumour infiltration. Later on, the follicles disappear and a diffuse pattern develops. The tumoural cells are mainly small to intermediate lymphoid cells, without pronounced pleomorphism, and interspersed with some large cells, immunoblastic or Sternberg-Reed-like.

Diffuse medium cells with nuclear polymorphism (pleomorphic small cell type). This type has a diffuse pattern and is composed predominantly of small- to intermediate-sized cells, with only slight variations in size, but more important variations in nuclear shape.

Mixed Cell Types

Lennert's lymphoma. Lymphoepithelioid lymphoma was described by Lennert as a special variant of Hodgkin's disease, but immunohistological and gene rearrangement studies further demonstrated the T-cell nature of the tumoural cells [33,34]. The predominant feature is the presence of small clusters of large epithelioid cells. The lymphoid cells are small- or medium-sized, and Sternberg-Reed-like cells are rare. This lymphoma must be differentiated from other NHLs with lymphoepithelioid content, such as Hodgkin's disease, lymphoplasmacytic lymphoma (lymphoplasmacytoid immunocytoma), angioimmunoblastic lymphadenopathy etc.

Angioimmunoblastic lymphadenopathy-like PTCL. This lesion, originally regarded as an abnormal immune reaction [35-37], was afterwards interpreted as a type of peripheral T-cell lymphoma called "IBL-like T-cell lymphoma" [38]. Gene rearrangement studies have confirmed this interpretation [39]. The striking feature is the large number of high endothelial postcapillary venules with an arborising pattern and thickened basement membranes. The tumour cells are large to intermediate and clusters of clear cells are sometimes seen.

Pleomorphous, Mixed-Cell and Large-Cell Types

These subtypes are diffuse tumours composed of variably-sized neoplastic cells with atypical nuclear configurations, variously described as convoluted, hyperconvoluted, cerebriform or multilobulated. Nuclei with one-sided multiple invaginations (jelly fish or banana bunch appearance) are frequently found. Two kinds of giant cells are recognised: Sternberg-Reed-like and cerebriform.
The tumour described as **Adult T-cell lymphoma/leukaemia** mostly belongs to this category: this aggressive, highly polymorphous PTCL is seen in southern Japan [40] and the Caribbean [41] as well as in migrants from these areas. It is associated with HTLV-1 retrovirus. The morphology of the leukaemic cells in the peripheral blood is characteristic in that their nuclei show strong lobulation and have been called "flower cells".
Immunoblastic T-cell lymphoma. This type is composed of large cells without pronounced polymorphism. Depending on the cytoplasm staining, the cells may have a basophilic or a clear cytoplasm. A variant is the **monomorphous medium-sized lymphoma** with a fairly abundant pale cytoplasm [42].
Large cell anaplastic type (Ki-1 positive) has been described elsewhere in this chapter.

Prognostic Value of Histological Classifications

To simplify therapeutic indications, the current histological classifications distinguish broad classes of behaviour. Thus, the WF recognises three prognostic groups (low, intermediate and high), whereas the KC only recognises two (low and high grades). But the predictive value of the intermediate group of the WF does not appear today to be different from that of the high grade [43]. Some rearrangements of the prognostic groups of these classifications have been shown to give a much better separation of the survival curves [44,45].

Good-Risk Histopathological Group

Good-risk B-cell NHLs are clinically indolent diseases with long median survival, but rarely curable. They were originally defined on the basis of the Rappaport classification as a group including nodular (follicular) and lymphocytic well-differentiated NHL. The existence of this good-risk group has been confirmed by many European studies showing differences between the subtypes of the low grade group of the KC according to the architectural pattern: within this low-grade group, the follicular (or follicular and diffuse) forms were shown to have a better prognosis that the diffuse forms [44-46]. Thus, this favourable group appears to be correctly defined by the follicular types B and C of the WF.

There are still some controversies about the prognosis of the lympho-plasmacytic subtype [45,47]. In the interpretation of survival in NHL, it appears necessary to exclude cases with chronic lymphocytic and Waldenstrom's macroglobulinaemia, which have their own prognostic factors and therapeutic strategies. On the other hand, many cases of lymphoplasmacytic/cytoid forms of the KC do not correspond to the low-grade group of the WF (subtype A) but rather to the intermediate-grade group (subtype F). Indeed, the lymphoplasmacytic type of the KC appears to be of poor prognosis [47].

The separation of a good-risk group within T-cell NHL is much more difficult. Although a low-grade group is distinguished in the updated KC, this distinction appears mainly based on morphological cellular features and, according to Suchi and Lennert, "does not necessarily reflect the grade of aggressiveness in their clinical behaviour" [12]. For instance, the presentation of the T-zone NHL in the updated KC (Table 1) as an entity having some degree of correspondence with follicular centroblastic-centrocytic does not implicate the same prognostic significance. The single confirmed good-risk T group, after exclusion of chronic T-cell leukaemias, is defined by cutaneous epidermotropic T-cell lymphomas: patients with these diseases may show skin involvement for long periods of time before frank tumour evolution occurs with involvement of other tissues.

Poor-Risk Histopathological Group

Aggressive B-cell NHLs are logically defined by the predominance of large (blastic) cells (more than 50%). Although the diffuse mixed and diffuse large cells (centroblastic diffuse) were included in the intermediate grade of the WF, this group appears now in many studies to have a poor prognosis, with no difference in survival from B-immunoblastic NHL. The predictability of the WF is improved with the shift of the subtype G (large cell corresponding to the centroblast type of KC) from intermediate grade to high grade [45]. Thus, the B-cell aggressive group is mainly defined by a diffuse pattern and a percentage of large (blastic) cells of more than 30%. Diffuse mixed (centroblastic-centrocytic, diffuse, large-cell) and diffuse large B-cell (centroblastic, diffuse), B-immunoblastic, B-lymphoblastic and Burkitt's are generally interpreted as NHL of aggressive histology. Follicular large cell (centroblastic, follicular) is also usually included is this group.

Among T NHLs, T-lymphoblastic is a highly aggressive lymphoma. But what about peripheral T-cell lymphomas? Despite their subclassification into many subtypes, data from Japan as from Europe and the U.S. indicate that all PTCLs have an aggressive natural history. Thus, it seems preferable to interpret all the non-epidermotropic PTCLs as aggressive lymphomas.

Intermediate-Risk Group

The definition of the intermediate-risk group obviously depends on the arrangement chosen for the good-risk and poor-risk groups. The intermediate-grade group of the original WF does not have a survival significantly different from the high grade [43]. An intermediate grade has been identified within the KC, according to the growth pattern, by separating low-grade diffuse types from the follicular types [45]. In the main, two entities belong to

this intermediate prognosis group: centrocytic diffuse, small-cell, (diffuse, intermediate lymphocytic differentiation and diffuse small-cleaved) and lymphoplasmocytic/cytoid [47]. Finally, the percentage of large blastic cells (greater than 20% or 30%?) may well be the critical factor in prognosis, but its evaluation is too subjective and hardly reproducible with the conventional histological analysis.
Nowadays, the predictive value of morphological classifications has some limitations: the improvement of chemotherapeutic treatment contributes to erasing the prognostic significance of the morphological subclassification of aggressive NHL [13,48]. On the other hand, the prognosis of NHL depends on many other factors, such as clinical stage, tumour mass, kinetic rate, performance status etc. In the coming years, classifications based on morphometric, kinetic and molecular criteria will probably become more important. For instance, some studies suggest that the proliferative rates of NHL as assessed by the Ki-67 antibody have clinical significance and may correlate with prognosis within a given subtype [49-52]. Prospective studies may show this kinetic information to have a prognostic value, independent of histology.

REFERENCES

1 Isaacson P and Wright DH: Extranodal malignant lymphoma arising from mucosa-associated lymphoid tissue. Cancer 1984 (53):2515-2524

2 Isaacson PG and Spencer J: Malignant lymphoma of mucosa-associated lymphoid tissue. Histopathology 1987 (11):445-447

3 Myrhre MJ and Isaacson PG: Primary B-cell gastric lymphoma - A reassessment of its histogenesis. J Pathol 1987 (152):1-11

4 Isaacson PG: Parafollicular B lymphocytes. Am J Clin Pathol 1988 (88):393

5 Hall PA, Jass RJ, Levison DA, Morson BA, Shepherd NA, Sobin NA and Stansfeld AG: Classification of primary gut lymphomas. Lancet 1988 (ii):958

6 Isaacson PG, O'Connor NTJ, Spencer J, Bevan DH, Connolly CE, Kirkham N, Pollock DJ, Wainscoat JS, Stein H and Mason DY: Malignant histiocytosis of the intestine: A T-cell lymphoma. Lancet 1986 (i):688-691

7 Berger F, Coiffier B, Bonneville C, Scoazec JY, Magaud JP and Bryon PA: Gastrointestinal lymphomas. Immunohistologic study of 23 cases. Am J Clin Pathol 1987 (88):707-719

8 Sheibani K, Burke JS, Swartz WG, Nademanee A and Winberg CD: Monocytoid B-Cell lymphoma. Clinicopathologic study of 21 cases of a unique type of low-grade lymphoma. Cancer 1988 (62):1531-1538

9 Sheibani K, Fritz RM, Winberg CD, Burke JS and Rappaport H: "Monocytoid" cells in reactive follicular hyperplasia with and without multifocal histiocytic reactions: an immunohistochemic study of 21 cases including suspected cases of toxoplasmic lymphadenitis. Am J Clin Pathol 1984 (81):453-458

10 Stein H, Lennert K, Mason DY, Liangu S and Ziegler A: Immature sinus histiocytes.Their identification as a novel B-cell population. Am J Pathol 1984 (117):44-52

11 Stein H, Mason DY and Gerdes J: The expression of the Hodgkin's disease associated antigen Ki1 in reactive and neoplastic lymphoid tissue: evidence that Reed-Sternberg cells and histiocytic malignancies are derived from activated lymphoid cells. Blood 1985 (66):848-858

12 Suchi T, Lennert K, Tu LY, Kikuchi M, Sato E, Stansfeld AG and Feller AC: Histopathology and immunohistochemistry of peripheral T-cell lymphomas: a proposal for their classification. J Clin Pathol 1987 (40):995-1015

13 Coiffier B, Bryon PA, Berger F, Archimbaud E, Ffrench M, Extra JM, Guyotat D, Fiere D, Gentilhomme O, Magaud JP, Blanc M, Peaud PY, Vuvan H and Viala JJ: Intensive and sequential combination chemotherapy for aggressive malignant lymphomas (protocol LNH 80). J Clin Oncol 1986 (4):147-153

14 Moller P, Moldenhauer G, Momburg F, Lämmier B, Eberlein-Gonska M, Kiesel S and Dörken B: Mediastinal lymphoma of clear cell type is a tumor corresponding to terminal steps of B-cell differentiation. Blood 1987 (69):1087-1095

15 Perrone T, Frizzera G and Rosai J: Mediastinal diffuse large-cell lymphoma with sclerosis. Am J Surg Pathol 1986 (10):176-191

16 Isaacson PG and Addis BJ: Lymphoma of the Thymus. In: Sarrazin, Vroussos, Vincent (eds) Thymic Tumors. Karger, Basle1989. pp 45-55

17 Harousseau JL, Andrieu JM, d'Agay MF and Tricot G: Diffuse large cell lymphoma with sclerosis localized to the mediastinum. A potentially curable clinicopathological entity. In: Sarrazin, Vroussos, Vincent (eds) Thymic Tumors. Karger, Basle 1989. pp 221-226

18 Chan JKC, Ng CS, Lau WH and Lo STH: Most nasal/nasopharyngeal lymphomas are peripheral T-cell neoplasms. Am J Surg Pathol 1987 (11):418-429

19 Jaffe E: The pathologic and clinical spectrum of post-thymic T-cell malignancies. Cancer Invest 1984 (2):413-426

20 Rilke F and Lennert K: A perspective of the Kiel classification in relation to other recent classifications of non-Hodgkin's lymphoma, with special reference to the Working Formulation. In: Lennert K (ed) Histopathology of Non-Hodgkin's Lymphomas (based on the Kiel classification). Springer-Verlag, Berlin Heidelberg New-York 1981. pp 112-118

21 Diebold J and Audouin J: The "Working Formulation of non-Hodgkin's lymphoma for clinical usage": a critical study. In: Sotto JJ, Vroussos C, Sotto MF, Vincent F (eds) Non Hodgkin's Lymphomas: New Techniques and Treatments. Karger, Basle 1985. pp 13-19

22 Nathwani BN and Winberg CD: Non-Hodgkin's lymphomas: an appraisal of the "Working Formulation" of non-Hodgkin's lymphomas for clinical usage. In: Sommers SC, Rosen PP (eds) Malignant Lymphomas. A Pathology Annual Monograph. Appleton-Century-Crofts, Norwalk 1983. pp 1-63

23 Stansfeld AG, Diebold J, Kapanci Y, Kelenyi G, Lennert K, Mioduszewska O, Noel H, Rilke F, Sundstrom C, Van Unik JAM and Wright DH:

Updated Kiel classification for lymphomas. Lancet 1988 (1):292-293

24 Krueger GRF, Medina JR, Klein HO, Konrads A, Zach J, Rister M et al: A new Working Formulation for non Hodgkin's lymphomas. A retrospective study of the new NCI classification proposal in comparison to the Rappaport and Kiel classifications. Cancer 1983 (52):833-840

25 Nanba K, Yamamoto H, Kamada N, Kikuchi M, Suchi T, Frizzera G, Berard CW, Shimamura K, Kaneko Y and Sakurai M: Agreement rates and American-Japanese pathologists. Comparability of a modified Working Formulation for non-Hodgkin's Lymphomas. An analysis of the cases collected for the fifth international workshop on chromosomes in leukemia-lymphoma. Cancer 1987 (59):1463-1469

26 Weisenburger DD, Nathwani BN, Diamond LW, Winberg CD and Rappaport H: Malignant lymphoma, intermediate lymphocytic type: A clinicopathologic study of 42 cases. Cancer 1981 (48):1415-1425

27 Weinsenburger DD, Kim H and Rappaport H: Mantle-zone lymphoma: A follicular variant of intermediate lymphocytic lymphoma. Cancer 1982 (49):1429-1438

28 Hui PK, Feller AC and Lennert K: High-grade non-Hodgkin's lymphoma of B-cell type. 1. Histopathology. Histopathology 1988 (12):127-143

29 Van der Putte SCJ, Schuurman HJ, Rademakers LHPM, Kluin PH and Van Unnik JAM: Malignant of follicle center cells with marked nuclear lobation. Virchows Arch (Cell Pathol) 1984 (46):93-107

30 Felman P, Bryon PA, Gentilhomme O, Magaud JP, Manel AM, Coiffier B and Lenoir G: Burkitt's lymphoma: multiparametric analysis of 55 cell lines with special reference to morphometry.In: Cavalli F, Bonadonna G and Rozenczweig M (eds) Malignant Lymphomas and Hodgkin's Disease: Experimental and Therapeutic Advances. Martinus Nijhoff, Boston 1985

31 Felman P, Bryon PA, Gentilhomme O, Magaud JP, Manel AM, Coiffier B and Lenoir G: Burkitt's lymphoma. Distinction of subgroups by morphometric analysis of the characteristics of 55 cell lines. Anal Quant Cytol Histol 1985 (7):275-282

32 Coiffier B, Berger F, Bryon PA and Magaud JP: T-cell lymphomas: immunologic, histologic, clinical, and therapeutic analysis of 63 cases. J Clin Oncol 1988 (6):1584-1589

33 Lennert K and Mestdagh J: Lymphogranulomatosen mit konstant hohem Epitheloidzellgehalt. Virchows Arch (Pathol Anat) 1968 (344):1-20

34 O'Connor NTJ, Feller AC, Wainscoat JS, et al: T-cell origin of Lennert's lymphoma. Brit J Haematol 1986 (64):521-528

35 Frizzera G, Moran EM and Rappaport H: Angioimmunoblastic lymphadenopathy with dysproteinemia. Lancet 1974 (i):1070-1073

36 Lukes RJ and Tindle BH: "Immunoblastic lymphadenopathy", a hyperimmune entity resembling Hodgkin's disease. N Engl J Med 1975 (292):1-8

37 Radszkiewicz T and Lennert K: Lymphogranulomatosis X. Klinisches Bild, Therapie und Prognose. Deutsch Med Wochenschr 1975 (100):1157-1163

38 Shimoyama M, Minato K, Saito H, et al: Immunoblastic lymphadenopathy (IBL)-like T-cell lymphoma. Jpn J Clin Oncol 1979 (9 Suppl):347-356

39 Weiss LM, Strickler JG, Dorfman RF, Horning SJ, Warnke RA and Sklar J: Clonal T-cell populations in angioimmunoblastic lymphadenopathy and angioimmunoblastic lymphadenopathy-like lymphoma. Am J Pathol 1986 (122):392-397

40 Uchiyama T, Yodoi J, Sagawa K, Tatasuki K and Uchino H: Adult T-cell leukemia: Clinical and hematological features of 17 cases. Blood 1977 (50):481-492

41 Catowski D, Greaves MF, Rose M, Galton DAG, Goolden AWG, McCluskey DR, White JM, Lampert I, Bourikas G, Ireland R, Brownell AI, Bridges JM, Blattner WA and Gallo RC: Adult T-cell lymphoma-leukaemia in blacks from the West Indies. Lancet 1982 (i):639-643

42 Watanabe S, Nakajima T, Shimosato Y, et al: T-cell malignancies: Subclassification and interelationship. Jpn J Clin Oncol 179 (9 Suppl):423-442

43 Simon RS, Durrleman S, Hoppe RT, Bonadonna G, Bloomfield CD, Rudders RA, Cheson BD and Berard CW: The non-Hodgkin lymphoma pathologic classification project. Long term follow-up of 1153 Patients with non-Hodgkin Lymphomas. An Int Med 1988 (109):939-945

44 De Wolf-Peeters C, Caillou B, Diebold J, Van Heerde P, Van Unnik JAM, Van der Oord JJ, Van Glabbeke M and Sommers R: Reproducibility and prognostic value of different non-Hodgkin's lymphoma classifications: Study based on the clinicopathologic relations found in the EORTC trial (20751). Eur J Cancer Clin Oncol 1985 (21):579-584

45 Nabholtz JM, Friedman S, Colin F and Guerrin J: Modification of Kiel and Working Formulation classifications for improved survival prediction in non-Hodgkin's lymphoma. J Clin Oncol 1987 (5):1634-1639

46 Meuge C, Hoerni B, Demascarel A, Durand M, Richaud P, Hoerni-Simon G, Chauvergne J and Lagarde C: Non-Hodgkin's malignant lymphomas:

Clinicopathologic correlations with the Kiel Classification. Retrospective analysis of a series of 274 cases. Eur J Cancer 1978 (14):587-592
47 Richards MA, Hall PA, Gregory WM, Dhaliwal HS, Stansfeld AG, Amess JAL and Lister TA: Lymphoplasmocytoid and small cell centrocytic non-Hodgkin's lymphoma - A retrospective analysis from St Bartholomew's Hospital 1972-1986. Hemat Oncol 1989 (7):19-35
48 Coiffier B, Gisselbrecht C, Herbrecht R, Tilly H, Bosly A and Brousse N: LNH-84 regimen: a multicenter study of intensive chemotherapy in 749 patients with aggressive malignant lymphoma. J Clin Oncol 1989 (in press)
49 Gerdes J, Dallenbach F and Lennert K: Growth fractions in malignant non-Hodgkin's lymphomas as determined in situ with the monoclonal antibody Ki-67. Hematol Oncol 1984 (2):365-371
50 Weiss LM, Strickler JG, Medeiros LJ, Gerdes J, Stein H and Warnke RA: Proliferative rates of non-Hodgkin's lymphomas as assessed by Ki-67 antibody. Hum Pathol 1987 (18):115-1159
51 Souchier C, Ffrench M, Berger F, Scoazec JY and PA Bryon: Image analysis applied to proliferating cells in malignant lymphoma. Cytometry 1988 (9):201-205
52 Grogan TM, Lippman SM, Spier CM, Slymen DJ, Rybski JA, Rangel CS, Richter LC and Miller TP: Independent prognostic significance of a nuclear proliferation antigen in diffuse large cell lymphomas as determined by the monoclonal antibody Ki-67. Blood 1988 (71):1157-1160

Management of Non-Hodgkin's Lymphomas: Conclusions of the First Intercity Meeting, 1986

Bertrand Coiffier [1], André Bosly [2], Federico Caligaris-Cappio [3], Christian Gisselbrecht [4], Catherine Patte [5], Michael Schaadt [6] and Michel Symann [7]

1 Haematology Service, Centre Hospitalier Lyon-Sud Pierre Bénite, Lyon, France
2 Cliniques Universitaires de Mont-Godinne, Yvoir, Belgium
3 Clinica Medica A, Università di Torino, Turin, Italy
4 Hôpital Saint-Louis, Paris, France
5 Institut Gustave Roussy, Villejuif, France
6 Medizinische Universitätsklinik, Köln, Federal Republic of Germany
7 Ludwig Institute for Cancer Research, Brussels Branch, Brussels, Belgium

On 15 December 1986 in Strasbourg (France) the first Intercity Meeting of the European School of Oncology was held with a survey of the current status of non-Hodgkin's lymphoma (NHL) management. The conclusions of this meeting are presented here. The Working Formulation for clinical use [1] (Table 1) is used throughout this paper.

Table 1. Working formulation of histologic types of non-Hodgkin's lymphomas [1]

Low grade	
A.	ML small lymphocytic
B.	ML follicular predominantly small cleaved cell
C.	ML follicular mixed, small cleaved and large cell
Intermediate grade	
D.	ML follicular predominantly large cell
E.	ML diffuse small cleaved cell
F.	ML diffuse mixed, small and large cell
G.	ML diffuse large cell
High grade	
H.	ML large cell, immunoblastic
I.	ML lymphoblastic
J.	ML small noncleaved cell
Miscellaneous	
	ML composite
	ML histiocytic
	ML unclassifiable

Reprinted with permission from Eur. J. Cancer Clin. Oncol., Vol. 23, No. 11, pp 1691-1695, 1987, Pergamon Press PLC

Follicular Low-Grade NHL

These lymphomas are characterised by the presence of a follicular pattern of infiltration of small cleaved cells or small and large cells. The percentage of large cells required to define low-grade NHL is still a matter of controversy [2]. The course is characterised by 3 phases: the first is marked by noticeable lymphadenopathies which do not seem to change with time; in the second phase they expand rapidly and symptoms can appear; in the third phase there is transformation of the low-grade NHL into a high-grade type resistant to therapy. The duration of each phase varies considerably from patient to patient. The major problems associated with these NHLs are the low frequency of truly localised forms, the impossibility of curing a large number of patients, the difficulty of obtaining a true complete remission (CR) and a constant mortality rate with a median survival of 6-8 years. Low survival is associated with such variables as age, bulky tumour, B symptoms (fever, sweats and weight loss) and increased lactate dehydrogenase (LDH) level [3]. Recently, the percentage of small non-cleaved cells and large non-cleaved cells at diagnosis has been negatively associated with survival and positively with histological progression [2].

Localised low-grade NHL can be cured by involved-field radiotherapy [3] and this treatment should be applied to all such patients. Advanced low-grade NHL remains a therapeutic challenge; the patients respond well at first to several regimens but continue to relapse and die. No significant difference between the various treatments have been documented in several randomised trials [4,5]; single drugs such as cyclophosphamide or chlorambucil produce the same results as polychemotherapy (CVP) with or without adriamycin. Some controversy persists as to whether achieving CR has any influence on survival.

Current recommendations for the treatment of these patients are difficult to point out. Some research groups advocate the "watch and wait" approach until progression [4], while others suggest that intensive chemotherapy should be attempted in some patients [6]. The optimal treatment is not known and should be sought by means of large cooperative trials wherein the widened recruitment could substantially reduce the time needed to obtain meaningful results. Questions which future studies should try to answer are: (a) Is there a group of patients in whom treatment could be delayed till progression? Would the absence of treatment be detrimental in terms of survival or percentage of patients who subsequently undergo histological progression? (b) Is the dose-response relationship which has been demonstrated in aggressive NHL also applicable to low-grade NHL? If so, what is (are) the best regimen(s)? (c) What role, if any, can be played by the new strategies such as interferon or intensification with bone marrow rescue? All of these questions are unanswered, the problem is to define how each particular type of case should be managed.

Paediatric Lymphomas

Childhood NHLs differ considerably from adult forms in that low and intermediate grade NHLs are rare in children; more than 90% of patients have lymphoblastic or small non-cleaved types, mostly Burkitt's. Nearly all young patients have widespread disease at time of diagnosis. In lymphoblastic lymphomas malignant cells are small, often convoluted, immature cells, usually of immature T-cell phenotype not very different from those observed in T-cell acute lymphoblastic leukaemia. Intensive combination chemotherapy (Table 2) has totally transformed their prognosis: a regimen such as the LSA_2-L_2 protocol can achieve a long-term disease-free survival rate of around 75% in disseminated disease [7].

Non-lymphoblastic lymphomas are of B-cell phenotype and are generally comprised of small non-cleaved cells, of Burkitt's or non-Burkitt's type. The disease generally originates in the gastrointestinal tract, abdominal cavity or Waldeyer's ring. Here too, intensive chemotherapy regimens have changed the prognosis: regimens such as the French LMB protocol [8] or the German BFM protocol [9] can produce a long-term survival rate of 60-70% for disseminated disease. For the rare localised NHLs, a long-term survival rate of 90% has been obtained with less intensive regimens.

Problems persist for the most aggressive presentations: patients with initial CNS involvement, especially when combined with marrow involvement, and those with extensive visceral involvement. Such patients fail to respond to intensive initial therapy. In cases with CNS involvement, high-dose methotrexate with folinic acid rescue or high-dose cytarabine permit some improvement [8]. In the remaining cases, intensification with bone marrow rescue offers some chance of long-term survival [10].

Aggressive Lymphomas

Major progress in the treatment of patients with aggressive NHL (intermediate and high grade) has been accomplished since 1975. The addition of adriamycin to the CVP regimen (cyclophosphamide, vincristine and prednisone), resulting in combinations such as the CHOP and BACOP regimens, has led to an improvement in CR rates, with a plateau in the survival curves. This suggests that long-term disease-free survival, and perhaps cure, is attainable [11]. The South West

Table 2. Drugs included in intensive chemotherapy regimens utilised in the treatment of non-Hodgkin's lymphomas and cited in the text

LSA_2-L_2 [7]:	induction:	CPM, VCR, MTX, DNR, Pred
	consolidation:	AraC, TG, Asp, MTX, BCNU
	maintenance:	TG, CPM, HU, DNR, MTX, BCNU, AraC, VCR
LMB [8]:	induction	CPM, VCR, Pred, MTX, ADR, AraC, Asp, CCNU, TG
	maintenance:	MTX, CPM, Pred, ADR, CCNU, AraC, TG, Asp
BFM [9]:	induction:	Pred, VCR, DNR, Asp
	consolidation:	CMP, AraC, MTX, MP
	maintenance:	MP, MTX, VCR, Pred
M-BACOD [13]:		Bleo, ADR, CPM, VCR, Dex
ProMACE-MOPP [14]:		CPM, ADR, VP16, Pred, NH_2, VCR, PCZ, MTX
MACOP-B [15]:		MTX, ADR, CPM, VCR, Bleo, Pred
LNH-80 [16]:	induction:	CPM, ADR, VCR, Bleo, mPred, MTX
	consolidation:	AraC, MTX, Asp
	intensification:	CPM, VM, Bleo, AraC, mPred
LNH-84:	induction:	CPM, ADR, VDS, Bleo, mPred, MTX
	consolidation:	AraC, MTX, Asp, VP16, IFM
	intensification:	CPM, VM, Bleo, AraC, mPred

ADR: doxorubicin, Asp: L-asparaginase, AraC: cytarabine, BCNU: carmustine, Bleo: bleomycin, CCNU: lomustine, CPM: cyclophosphamide, Dex: dexamethasone, DNR: daunorubicin, HU: hydroxyurea, IFM: ifosfamide, MP: mercaptopurine, mPred: methylprednisolone, MTX: methotrexate, NH_2: mechlorethamine, PCZ: procarbazine, Pred: prednisone, TG: thioguanine, VCR: vincristine, VDS: vindesine, VM: teniposide, VP16: etoposide

Oncology Group has recently reported a more than 10 year follow up of patients treated by CHOP, indicating that 30% of the patients were probably cured [12].

These results have been dramatically improved by intensive combination chemotherapy (Table 2). Regimens such as M-BACOD [13], ProMACE-MOPP [14], MACOP-B [15] and LNH-80 [16] have been associated with 60-80% CR rates. The increase in CR rates is associated with a decrease in relapse rate, and thus 50-70% of patients survived 3 years or longer. However, long-term results (5 or 10 years of follow up) are not available for all these intensive regimens, and thus the advantage in terms of survival is not definitively known. A major difficulty in comparing these treatments is that they differ with respect to eligibility criteria (prior therapy, stage, performance status, morphological subtypes) and the incidence of known prognostic factors. For example, the M/m-BACOD study clearly demonstrates the importance of performance status, tumour bulk and the number of extranodal sites of disease [17]; but marrow involvement was present in only 10% of cases instead of 25-30% in major studies. The influence of age on response and survival is also well documented [18], but the median age and the number of patients over 60 years differ from one study to the other. A prognostic index was constructed by Shipp et al. [17], based on performance status, the diameter of the largest mass and the number of extranodal sites of disease, which divided the patients into 3 groups with predicted 5-year survival rates of 68, 55 and 24%, respectively. In the LNH-80 regimen we also found these variables to be significant but marrow involvement proved to be the major prognostic factor, both in terms of response and survival. By applying the Shipp's index, we obtained 5-year survival rates of 77, 73 and 52%, respectively [19]. Multicentre randomised studies are currently in progress in the US and Europe to define the best therapeutic regimen.

Some issues are still a matter of debate. (a) Should lymphoblastic NHL and small noncleaved cell NHL in adults be treated like other aggressive NHLs? The answer is that true lymphoblastic T-cell NHL in the young adult is similar to T-cell acute lymphoblastic leukaemia, especially if the marrow is involved, and should therefore be treated as T-cell acute lymphoblastic leukaemia. Nonconvoluted non-Burkitt lymphoblastic NHLs, as defined by the Kiel classification, are mostly unclassified NHLs and should be treated as adult aggressive NHLs. Small non-cleaved cell NHLs of Burkitt's or non-Burkitt's type are very aggressive NHLs in the adult and require intensive regimens such as LNH-80 or intensive paediatric regimens. (b) What duration of chemotherapy is needed? The MACOP-B regimen clearly demonstrates that chemotherapy could be limited if it is intensive. We are currently testing the need for a final intensification in the LNH-84 protocol, in a multicentrre randomised study based on the LNH-80 regimen. Preliminary results based on the first 600 patients will be published soon. (c) Are peripheral T-cell NHLs (PTCLs) different from other aggressive NHLs? This question has rarely been addressed, possibly because PTCLs were rarely recognised in the past and hence few such patients were included in protocols. PTCLs do not readily fit in our present morphological classifications and thus are frequently assigned to the unclassified group or are not diagnosed as NHL but as related disease such as angioimmunoblastic lymphadenopathy [20] or Hodgkin's disease. PTCL patients had the worst prognosis out of all the groups studied in our LNH-80 protocol [19]: median survival was only 14 months for PTCL and not reached for B-cell NHL or untyped NHL. This poor prognosis is related to either death during the induction chemotherapy, failure to respond or early relapses. However, in a non-randomised study of 50 PTCL patients, the LNH-80 regimen yielded the best survival figure [21]. (d) What is the place, if any, of radiotherapy in aggressive NHL? Clearly, aggressive NHLs are not a localised disease, even in cases with a localised presentation. Previous radiotherapy protocols for stage I or II patients have shown that relapses do not occur at the initial site of the disease [22]. Adjuvant chemotherapy after radiotherapy was proven to be indispensable. Results obtained using chemotherapy alone were found as good as those obtained with the chemotherapy-radiotherapy combination [23]. Radiotherapy may remain useful for CNS localisations or as adjuvant therapy in bulky tumours, although this is debatable.

Salvage Therapy

Twenty to 30% of the patients with an aggressive NHL failed to respond to chemotherapy and 20-30% of those who did respond relapsed. Thus, 30-40% of the patients need salvage therapy. No satisfactory universal chemotherapy is widely accepted and no standard recommendation exists for salvage therapy. The problem is that, because of the acquired multidrug resistance, patients who fail to respond to initial chemotherapy rarely respond to other treatments. Two solutions have been proposed: alternative regimens with non-cross-resistant drugs, or increased dosage of the drugs. Several alternative regimens have been described during the last 5 years, but very few display the characteristics of a good salvage regimen such as a CR rate of 50%; a relapse rate of less than 20%; no major toxicity, and at least 40% of patients still alive at least 2 years after salvage. The most effective regimen employed ifosfamide, etoposide, methylgag and methotrexate [24] but did not meet these criteria: only 20% of the patients were alive 2 years post salvage. Mitoxantrone may have a crucial part to play in this aspect of lymphoma treatment [25].

Increased drug dosage is feasible if followed by rescue by autologous bone marrow reinjection (ABMR). ABMR has been tested with some success in paediatric and adult patients [10,26]. CR was obtained in 40% of the patients, with half of them relapsing during the first year, resulting in a less than 25% 2-year survival. Several problems still prevent complete assessment of the merits of this type of therapy. (a) The inability to obtain complete responses in the majority of patients with refractory NHL is the major factor limiting successful ABMR treatment. (b) The possible reinfusion of lymphoma cells is not a real problem, even with unpurged marrow, as indicated by the similar results obtained by the Seattle group with syngenic, allogenic or autologous bone marrow cells. (c) The nature of the ablative chemotherapy or radio-chemotherapy before marrow rescue needs to be stated precisely. One possible alternative would be to perform early consolidation with ABMR in high-risk patients at the first CR. This possibility will be tested in our LNH-87 protocol.

The past decade has witnessed major progress in the treatment of NHL with more and more patients surviving at least 5 years who are possibly cured. But considerable work is necessary in order to attain a cure rate of at least 75%. The hardest part remains to be worked out and the challenge of the future can only be met by initiating large prospective cooperative trials.

REFERENCES

1 The National Cancer Institute sponsored study of classifications of non-Hodgkin's lymphomas: summary and description of a Working Formulation for clinical use. The non-Hodgkin's lymphoma pathologic classification project. Cancer 1982 (49):2112-2135

2 Nathwani BN, Metter GE, Miller TP et al: What should be the morphologic criteria for the subdivision of follicular lymphomas? Blood 1986 (68):837-845

3 Gospodarowicz MK, Bush RS, Brown TC, Chua T: Prognostic factors in nodular lymphomas: a multivariate analysis based on the Princess Margaret Hospital experience. Int J Radiat Oncol Biol Phys 1984 (10):489-497

4 Rosenberg SA: The low grade non-Hodgkin's lymphomas: challenges and opportunities. J Clin Oncol 1985 (102):596-602

5 Ezdinli EZ, Anderson JR, Melvin F, Glick JH, Davis TE, O'Connell MJ: Moderate versus aggressive chemotherapy of nodular lymphocytic poorly differentiated lymphoma. J Clin Oncol 1985 (3):769-775

6 Cheson BD, Wittes RE, Friedman MA: Low-grade non-Hodgkin's lymphomas revisited. Cancer Treat Rep 1986 (70):1051-1054

7 Anderson JR, Wilson JF, Jenkin RDT et al: Childhood non-Hodgkin's lymphomas. The results of a randomised therapeutic trial comparing a 4-drug regimen (COMP) with a 10-drug regimen (LSA_2-L_2). N Engl J Med 1983 (308):559-565

8 Patte C, Philip T, Rodary C et al: Improved survival rate in children with stage III and IV B cell non-Hodgkin's lymphoma and leukemia using multi-agent chemotherapy. Results of a study of 114 children from the French Pediatric Oncology Society. J Clin Oncol 1986 (4):1219-1226

9 Müller-Weihrich S, Henze G, Odenwald E, Riehm H: BFM trials for childhood non-Hodgkin's lymphomas. In: Cavalli F, Bonadonna G, Rozencweig M (eds) Malignant Lymphomas and Hodgkin's Disease: Experimental and Therapeutic Advances. Martinus Nijhoff, Boston 1985 pp 633-642

10 Hartmann O, Pein F, Beaujean F et al: High dose polychemotherapy with autologous bone marrow transplantation in children with relapsed lymphomas. J Clin Oncol 1984 (2):979-985

11 Armitage JO, Fyfe MAE, Lewis J: Long-term remission durability and functional status of patients treated for diffuse histiocytic lymphoma with the CHOP regimen. J Clin Oncol 1984 (2):889-902

12 Coltman CA, Dahlberg S, Jones SE et al: CHOP is curative in thirty per cent of patients with diffuse large cell lymphoma: a twelve year SWOG follow-up. Proc ASCO 1986 (5):774

13 Skarin AT, Canellos GP, Rosenthal D et al: Improved prognosis of diffuse histiocytic and undifferentiated lymphoma by use of high dose methotrexate alternating with standard agents (M-BACOD). J Clin Oncol 1983 (1):91-98

14 Fisher RI, DeVita VT, Hubbard SM et al: Diffuse aggressive lymphomas: increased survival after alternating flexible sequences of ProMACE and MOPP chemotherapy. Ann Intern Med 1983 (98):304-309

15 Klimo P, Connors JM: MACOP-B chemotherapy for the treatment of diffuse large-cell lymphomas. Ann Intern Med 1985 (102):596-602

16 Coiffier B, Bryon PA, Berger F et al: Intensive and sequential combination chemotherapy for aggressive malignant lymphomas protocol (LNH-80). J Clin Oncol 1986 (4):147-153

17 Shipp MA, Harrington DP, Klatt MM et al: Identification of prognostic subgroups of patients with large-cell lymphoma treated with m-BACOD or M-BACOD. Ann Intern Med 1986 (4):757-765

18 Dixon DO, Neilan B, Jones SE et al: Effect of age on therapeutic outcome in advanced diffuse histiocytic lymphoma. The Southwest Oncology Group experience. J Clin Oncol 1986 (4):295-305

19 Coiffier B, Sebban C, French M et al: Aggressive lymphomas treated by intensive chemotherapy: updated results of the LNH-80 protocol with a median follow-up of 52 months. Blood 1987 (5):1394-1399

20 Wanatabe S, Sato Y, Shimoyama M, Minato K, Shimosato Y: Immunoblastic lymphadenopathy, angioimmunoblastic lymphadenopathy, and IBL-like T-cell lymphoma. A spectrum of T-cell neoplasia. Cancer 1986 (58):2224-2232

21 Coiffier B, Berger F, Bryon PA, Magaud JP: Peripheral T-cell lymphomas: immunologic, histologic, clinical, and therapeutic analysis in 50 patients. Proc Am Soc Hematol 1986 (68):826

22 Kaminski MS, Coleman N, Colby TV, Cox RS, Rosenberg SA: Factors predicting survival in adults with stage I and II large-cell lymphoma treated with primary radiation therapy. Ann Intern Med 1986 (104):747-756

23 Cabanillas F: Chemotherapy as definitive treatment of stage I-II large cell and diffuse mixed lymphomas. Hematol Oncol 1985 (3):25-31

24 Cabanillas F, Hagemeiter FB, McLaughlin P et al: Results of MIME salvage regimen for recurrent or refractory lymphoma. J Clin Oncol 1987 (5):398-406

25 Rivkin SE, Peterson BA, Jones SE: Novanrone (mitoxantrone) in the therapy of non-Hodgkin's lymphoma: a phase II study. Protocol 3-46. Data on file, Lederle Laboratories

26 Armitage JO, Jagannath S, Spitzer G et al: High dose therapy and autologous marrow transplantation as salvage treatment for patients with diffuse large cell lymphoma. Eur J Cancer Clin Oncol 1986 (22):871-877

Management of Non-Hodgkin's Lymphomas in Elderly Patients: Conclusions of the Second Intercity Meeting, 1987

Vittoria Zagonel [1], Antonino Carbone [2], Sandor Kerpel-Fronius [3], Rolf Kuse [4], Svetislav Jelic [5], Heinz Huber [6], Umberto Tirelli [1], Heinz Ludwig [7], Stojan Plesnicar [8] and Silvio Monfardini [1]
with the collaboration of Reto Obrist [9], Giuseppe Cartei [10], Mauro Gaetano Trovò [11], Ivan Koza [12] and Marianne Engelhard [13]

1 Division of Medical Oncology, Centro di Riferimento Oncologico, Aviano, Italy
2 Division of Pathology, Centro di Riferimento Oncologico, Aviano, Italy
3 Department of Clinical Research, National Institute of Oncology, Budapest, Hungary
4 Department of Haematology, Allgemeines Krankenhaus St Georg, Hamburg, Federal Republic of Germany
5 Institute of Oncology and Radiology, Belgrade, Yugoslavia
6 Department of Internal Medicine, University Hospital, Innsbruck, Austria
7 II Medizinische Universitäts Klinik, Allgemeines Krankenhaus der Stadt Wien, Vienna, Austria
8 Chair of Oncology and Radiotherapy, University E. Kardelj, Ljubljana, Yugoslavia
9 Division of Oncology, Department of Internal Medicine, University Kantonsspital, Basle, Switzerland
10 Division of Medical Oncology, Ospedale Civile, Udine, Italy
11 Division of Radiotherapy, Centro di Riferimento Oncologico, Aviano, Italy
12 Department of Chemotherapy, Institute of Clinical Oncology, Bratislava, Czechoslovakia
13 Division of Haematology, Medizinische Klinik, University of Essen, Essen, Federal Republic of Germany

The occurrence of malignant non-Hodgkin's lymphomas (NHL) in *elderly* patients is a clinical condition probably requiring a specific therapeutic approach. This issue is, however, quite controversial, since it has only recently been brought to the attention of medical oncologists and haematologists: the few available studies in the literature provide rather conflicting results.
In order to examine therapeutic approaches, results and open problems, as well as the frequency and distribution of histological types in NHL of the elderly, a one-day meeting of clinical oncologists from the geographical area of Central Europe was organised in Vienna on 13th July, 1987, by the European School of Oncology. The conclusions of this second Intercity Meeting on non-Hodgkin's lymphomas, with emphasis on the elderly, are presented in this paper.

Pathological Features

The analysis of the frequency and distribution of the histological types of NHL in old age was mainly focused on providing possible clinico-pathological bases for further consideration in the management of NHL in the elderly. Whenever possible, the terminology of the Working Formulation (1982) was used as a means of translation among all classification systems for NHL [1].
The main difficulties encountered by this analysis were attributed to the fact that elderly patients are usually excluded from clinical trials [2]. As a consequence, pathological data concerning NHL of the elderly are scarce and fragmentary and also usually reported in one of the main classifications without mentioning the equivalent terms of the Working Formulation. This work could be carried out by analysing some of the major series published which contain tabular data or graphs concerning the frequency of NHL, together with the distribution of their histologi-

cal subtypes in old age and by a revision of a few recent papers specifically dealing with NHL of the elderly [3-10] (Table 1). Selected information on a series of 280 NHL patients consecutively observed during a 3-year period at the Division of Pathology of the Centro di Riferimento Oncologico of Aviano from June 1984 to May 1987 was also presented at this meeting to compare the pathological characteristics of 76 cases older than 70 years with those of 204 patients under 70 (Table 2). The salient points of this analysis, as well as the aforementioned series, show that elderly patients aged 65 years or more constitute a relevant proportion of all patients with NHL at a percentage varying from 17 to 34%. According to the Slovenian tumour registry of the Institute of Oncology of Ljubljana, 29% of patients over 70 with non-Hodgkin's lymphomas were reported in 1983. In the series observed at the Centro di Riferimento Oncologico of Aviano, 27.2% (76/280) of the patients were aged 70 years or older. In all these series the diffuse pattern was observed more frequently and the diffuse histiocytic, according to the Rappaport classification, was the most frequent histotype, ranging from 26 to 37%. Most of the NHLs observed at the Centro di Riferimento Oncologico of Aviano were of intermediate- (50%) or high-grade (21.7%) malignancy. This information confirmed the results of a previous experience at the same centre where intermediate and high grade histology also accounted for the majority of cases (84%) [8]. However, the frequency of intermediate and high grade histology among elderly patients did not differ from that observed in younger patients (Table 2). On the other hand, low-grade histotypes and follicular growth patterns are less frequently represented in the elderly group, as recently reported by Otter et al. in a large case series in The Netherlands [11].

Initial extranodal presentation and/or extranodal diffusion at onset were found not to be uncommon (47.4%) in the case series analysed at the Centro di Riferimento Oncologico of Aviano from 1984 to 1987. The same experience was reported through an analysis of the results performed at the Institute of Belgrade. Besides clinico-pathological features, some aspects of cellular and humoural immunological response in elderly patients were considered at the Division of Medical Oncology of the Udine General Hospital. In 42 patients with untreated non-Hodgkin's lymphomas an immunological study was undertaken, and results were evaluated according to age (from 50 to 84 years). The group of 14 patients over 70 years showed a statistical decrease of total T-cells (38.1%), of T-helper (H) (42.7%) and T-suppressor (S) subpopulations, the H/S ratio being unaffected. The B lymphocytes were also reduced (30%) in this group without significance, whilst serum IgA and IgM levels were significantly raised (71.8% and 80.7%, respectively).

Table 1. Frequency of NHL in old age

Authors	References	Patients aged ≥ 60 yrs	≥65 yrs	≥70 yrs	≥80 yrs
Jones 1973	[3]		17.7%		
Patchefsky 1974	[4]	38.5%			
Nathwani 1978	[5]	38.0%			
Anderson 1982	[6]	19.9%			
Mead 1984	[7]		19.0%		
Carbone 1986	[8]		27.0%		
Hoerni 1987	[9]				5.4%
Kuse 1987	[20]	52.0%			
Otter 1987	[11]			34.0%	

Table 2. Age and distribution of 229 patients* in the 10 subtypes of the WF classified at the Centro di Riferimento Oncologico of Aviano from 1984 to 1987

Group WF	<70 yrs	%	≥ 70 yrs	%	Total	%
A	24	14.2	10	16.7	34	14.8
B	6	3.6	3	5.0	9	3.9
C	14	8.3	4	6.7	18	7.8
Low Grade	44	26.1	17	28.4	61	26.6
D	9	5.3	2	3.3	11	4.8
E	12	7.1	5	8.3	17	7.4
F	34	20.1	15	25.0	49	21.4
G	21	12.4	8	13.3	29	12.7
Intermediate	76	44.9	30	49.9	106	46.3
H	36	21.3	10	16.7	46	20.1
I	7	4.1	2	3.3	9	3.9
J	6	3.6	1	1.7	7	3.1
High Grade	49	29.0	13	21.7	62	27.1

* Out of 280 consecutive cases 18 unclassified and 33 classified as miscellaneous

Pharmacology of Antitumour Drugs in Elderly Patients

The administration of antitumour agents to elderly patients should take into account that both the tissue tolerance and the pharmacokinetics might be altered by age. Unfortunately, not very much information is available on this subject. For this reason, a part of this meeting was specifically addressed to this point.

In Europe, people over 65 make up 10-12% of the population, but consume about 33% of the drug supply. The incidence of adverse drug reactions is rather high, generally more than 20%. Old people are usually treated parallelly for various chronic illnesses, mostly with multiple-drug therapies using diuretics, beta-blockers, analgesics, tranquillisers, hypnotics, etc. Obviously, the chances of interaction of cytostatics with other agents administered concomitantly are much higher in this age group. It may so happen that the activity of some antitumour drugs is potentiated or decreased through the action on absorption, distribution, excretion and metabolism of other drugs, or vice versa.

Although procarbazine should be considered as an extreme example, it might help to put the complexity of the problem into proper perspective. The drug is first converted by microsomal enzymes into active intermediates, which in turn are further metabolised to inactive metabolites by the same enzyme system. Since the former process seems to be of major importance, pretreatment with phenobarbital leads to increased concentration of active metabolites with a consequent increase in the effectiveness of therapy. At the same time, procarbazine inhibits the metabolic inactivation of barbiturates, thus prolonging their action [12,13]. Finally, procarbazine, being a monoamine oxidase inhibitor, sensitises patients to the ingestion of tyramine and to drugs that are degraded by this enzyme [14]. Unfortunately, the problem is further complicated by the known poor compliance in some 60% of the aged patients.

Altered organ sensitivity to drugs, especially the age-dependent decrease in the number of stem cells in the bone marrow [15], seems to be the crucial factor, according to broad clinical experience, in determining the degree of tolerance of patients to cytostatic agents in general. The higher vulnerability of the lungs to bleomycin in geriatric cases is also well known [16]. Besides these tolerability changes in the target organs, several physiological alterations result in the modification of the pharmacokinetic behaviour of drugs, which creates an additional source of toxicity in the elderly: 1) altered volume of distribution, due to loss of some 30% of cells from the tissues compensated by fat deposition and increased water content; 2) decreased plasma protein concentration; 3) diminished blood supply to the organs; 4) decreased hepatic metabolism and biliary excretion due to liver atrophy; 5) diminished renal excretion, due to loss of about 30% of the nephrons; 6) slower drug absorption, even if it is quantitatively generally adequate. From all these biliary and especially age-related changes, a diminished renal clearance [17] might frequently lead to serious adverse drug effects by significantly prolonging drug elimination, with the consequent increase in drug exposure time. At present, methotrexate is the only example for which an age-dependent decrease of renal elimination associated with increased toxicity has been clearly indicated, both clinically and pharmacokinetically [18-21]. On the basis of broad clinical experience, it seems that an elevated serum bilirubin level, but not the increase of serum transaminase, alkaline phosphatase and gamma-glutamyltranspeptidase activities, is associated with clinically significant changes of drug toxicity [22]. It would be more promising to look for correlations between hepatic function and drug toxicity in cancer patients, using tests that more faithfully reflect liver excretory and drug metabolising activity, such as indocyanine green and bromsulphalein retention, aminopyrene elimination, etc.

For the majority of antitumour drugs, pharmacokinetic data in patients over 70 are not available. As long as these results are missing, one can only extrapolate from the pharmacokinetic properties of anticancer agents described in adult patients with normal and abnormal organ functions, as well as from the known age-related pharmacokinetic changes elaborated above. Dose reduction strategy should be primarily planned considering the age-dependent decrease of renal clearance. Unfortunately, linear relationships between drug elimination and renal function rarely exist, primarily because most of the drugs are eliminated from the body by several pathways. One may only advocate making a 25% dose reduction if the creatinine clearance is moderately changed; 50% or higher decrease of the dose should be introduced only if the clearance is diminished to less than 20-25% of the normal value. Among the drugs used frequently for the treatment of malignant lymphomas, the following are candidates for dose adjustments in the presence of kidney troubles: 1) methotrexate, which is eliminated unchanged up to 90% in the urine [21,23,24]; 2) bleomycin, of which approximately half is excreted unchanged via the urine [20,23]; 3) cyclophosphamide, in which case kidney damage leads to elevated levels both of the parent compound and the active biotransformation products [25,26]; 4) DTIC, which is eliminated unchanged up to 50% by the kidney [27]; 5) from the epipodophyllotoxins the renal elimination of etoposide, but not teniposide, might be changed considering that about 23 to 45% of the former, but only up to 10% of the latter, is cleared unchanged by this route. However, no cases have been reported yet showing increased toxicity in the presence of kidney damage [27].

Dose reduction in the case of bile flow obstruction should be considered when using anthracyclines and vinca alkaloids: 1) up to about 50% of the various anthracycline derivatives are cleared unchanged, or in the form of active metabolites, through the biliary tract, thus it might be prudent to decrease the dose by 50% of all anthracycline analogues if the serum bilirubin level is between 1.2-3 mg% (20-52μmol/l), as was recommended originally for adriamycin by Benjamin and coworkers [29]. A decreased adriamycin early clearance was observed in the elderly by Robert and Hoerni [30], however, the functional implication of this finding remains obscure; 2) much less plasma level data exists for the vinca alkaloids, since easily applied chromatographic methods have become available only recently. As approximately half of the dose of both vincristine and vinblastine is excreted in the bile, a dose reduction similar to that recommended for the anthracyclines seems to be a prudent approach [31].

In conclusion, it is evident that carefully planned pharmacokinetic studies are needed in the elderly for the rational development of drug schedules that maintain a high therapeutic activity with acceptable toxicity. For the time being, an initial 25% dose reduction, followed by a careful individual evaluation of the tolerable dose, seems to be a reasonably cautious approach in the case of myelotoxic agents and bleomycin, considering the diminished tissue tolerance and altered pharmacokinetic parameters in the aged population. Further dose reduction should be made only if appropriate tests reveal serious impairment of the renal and/or biliary excretion, which is usually the consequence of allied diseases.

Treatment and Results

Not very much information is available at the present time on the results of treatment of NHL in elderly patients. Some authors consider 70 years to be the age limit, others 65. Median age of the considered population is sometimes not even reported. This makes a comparison between the different series very difficult. In this meeting, the analysis was restricted to patients of 70 years or more.

All data provided by the invited participants from Germany, Austria, Italy, Yugoslavia, Czechoslovakia and Switzerland were, thus, uniformly limited to patients for whom the breaking point was 70 years of age from 1980 to 1984. In almost all series reported at this meeting, a retrospective evaluation was mainly conducted in the effort of acquiring specific information on clinical characteristics at presentation, response to treatment, toxicity, and survival in this age population. Results of specific controlled studies worldwide are, in fact, not available at the moment. On the other hand, it is well known that, usually, only a minority of elderly patients are clinically eligible for research protocols [2].

The therapeutic approach was almost uniform among participating institutions. Local or large field radiotherapy alone ± combination chemotherapy was delivered to patients with stage I-II and high-grade histology, while patients with stage III and IV unfavourable lymphomas were treated with CHOP (cyclophosphamide, adriamycin, vincristine and prednisone), or CHOP-like regimens. Patients with a favourable histology were treated according to the various therapeutic options available today (single agents, combination chemotherapy, radiotherapy).

The experience of the St. Georg General Hospital of Hamburg from 1980 to 1984 consisted of 64 patients of ≥70 years of age with low-grade malignant lymphoma whose projected survival at 5 years (48%) did not significantly differ from that of 72 patients aged under 70 (60%). In the same period, the survival probability of 37 patients aged ≥70 years with high-grade histology at 5 years compared to that of 80 patients under 70, was practically equivalent (55% vs 60%). Only one patient died from toxicity. No dose-intensity analysis was available, but most elderly patients started treatment with a dose reduction of about one third of the standard projected dose.

The other German/Austrian group (Kiel Lymphoma Study Group) was able to study retrospectively an impressive number of patients with non-Hodgkin's lymphomas collected from 1975 to 1980 in a prospective multicentre observation study (follow-up period 1981-1985) conducted with the collaboration of a number of German and Austrian hospitals [32]. Of 782 NHLs of low-grade malignancy and 342 of high-grade malignancy, 187 (24%) and 86 (25%), respectively, were observed in patients over 70. The median survival for high-grade patients was low and similar in both groups (17 and 14 months, respectively). The complete-response (CR) rate was only 35% in patients over 70 and 45% in younger patients. It may be worth recalling that conventional chemotherapy and not intensive "second and third generation" chemotherapy (e.g., ProMACE-MOPP, ProMACE-CytaBOM, MACOP-B) was applied. Patients were also treated in internal medicine departments of general hospitals as well as haematology and medical oncology departments. Patients under 70 with low-grade lymphomas had a consistently better median survival (60 months) than those over 70 (31 months). Toxic death was equally represented in both age groups, afflicting 46 (5.4%) of the 854 cases younger than 70 and 12 (4.4%) of the 273 cases older than 70. No detailed analysis of different regimens used, nor dose-intensity analysis, were available, as the cases had been previously assembled with the primary goal of a uniform pathological analysis.

The analysis performed at the Institute of Oncology of Belgrade was based on the retrospective evaluation of 50 patients of 70 years or older, observed from 1981 to 1985. This report emphasised the fact that staging procedures such as bone marrow biopsy, lymphangiogram and abdominal CT scan could be carried out less extensively than in younger patients. Elderly patients were probably judged unsuitable for time-consuming treatments, with the tendency to stop treatment early, irrespective of response or socioeconomic status. However, patients from urban and suburban areas were less frequently lost to follow up compared to those coming from rural areas. Overall CR rate to chemotherapy was 47% with a higher response rate in patients with low-grade, compared to those with high- and intermediate-grade histology. Overall survival of patients treated with chemotherapy at 12 months was 42%.

The experience of the Institute of Clinical Oncology of Bratislava was based on 32 patients with a median age of 72 years (range 70-89 years) of a predominantly unfavourable type. Although CR was obtained in 40% of cases and median survival of high-grade complete responders was 34 months, significant comorbidity (heart, lung and liver) and fulminant infection were thought to be a much more serious problem than in younger patients. These patients required longer hospitalisation and close follow up in the clinic and were afflicted by frequent psychological changes.

At the Centro di Riferimento Oncologico of Aviano a first retrospective clinico-pathological study was conducted on 50 patients of 65 years or older seen between 1975 and 1981, as reported in the first part of this paper. Between August 1979 and September 1984, prospective studies using specifically devised chemotherapy regimens were carried out with the aim of reducing the significant toxicity associated with aggressive treatments observed in the first retrospective study [33] and in those of others [10,34]. Seventy-one consecutive unselected elderly patients (median age 76, range 70-85) entered 2 consecutive prospective trials, the former with the epipodophyllotoxin derivative teniposide 100 mg/m^2 i.v. weekly (42 patients), the latter with etoposide and prednimustine, both 100 mg/m^2 p.o. for 5 days once every 3 weeks (29 patients). Eighty-seven per cent were stages III and IV, 72% were intermediate and high grade, according to the Working Formulation. Those patients with low-grade stage III and IV had systemic symptoms. The results of these consecutive studies were put together because of the similarity of the treatments employed and because of the patient characteristics [35,36]. The results obtained in the 15 patients with diffuse histiocytic lymphoma (DHL) subtype (53% CR) compare favourably with those obtained by other authors in elderly patients [34] with CHOP (45% CR), but with a significantly lower toxicity. The 3-year survival of Italian "healthy" persons with a median age of 75 years was similar to that of these previously untreated elderly patients who achieved CR (60% vs 57%). The conclusions of this Italian group were as follows: 1) elderly patients present mostly with intermediate and high-grade NHL; 2) the CR rate achieved in 45 consecutive untreated elderly patients ($\geq$ 70 years, median age 76) with NHL of unfavourable prognosis treated with epipodophyllotoxins $\pm$ prednimustine is comparable to that observed by other authors [34] in patients treated with CHOP; 3) treatment-related toxicity (3% deaths) observed in this population of unselected elderly patients compares favourably with the CHOP-related toxicity (30% deaths) observed in a population of elderly patients of similar median age reported by other authors [34].

During the meeting, the results of a retrospective EORTC Lymphoma Group survey proposed by members of the Institute of Aviano were also mentioned. This study was undertaken at 50 different European institutes, with the aim of evaluating the incidence and the outcome of NHL in the elderly patients observed during 1984. Thus far, 127 patients (median age 77, range 70-90) had been identified at 12 institutes. Among the 64 patients treated with aggressive treatments (AT), defined as chemotherapy regimens with >3 drugs or combined treatments, treatment-related deaths had occurred in 9 patients (14%) and severe toxicity (grades III-IV according to WHO) in an additional 16 patients (25%). On the other hand, among the 57 patients treated with conservative treatments (CT), including local radiotherapy or chemotherapy regimens with $\leq$2 drugs, there was no lethal toxicity, and severe toxicity was observed in only 3 patients (6%). This difference was highly significant ($p < 0.001$). The CR rate was 30% in patients treated with AT and 33% in patients treated with CT [36].

Discussion and Conclusions

Is the occurrence of malignant lymphomas in elderly patients a clinical condition requiring specific therapeutic considerations? This issue is quite controversial with conflicting results deriving from the few studies reported in the literature.

Armitage and Potter evaluated retrospectively the outcome of 20 patients aged 70 years or older with diffuse histiocytic lymphoma (DHL) and predominantly (75%) advanced-stage disease treated with the CHOP regimen at full doses [34]. Although the complete remission rate observed was not significantly different from that of a younger group of patients with DHL treated concurrently with CHOP, 30% treatment-related deaths occurred, the major factor being sepsis. On the other hand, Miller and Jones reported a series of 11 patients older than 65 years with clinically localised NHL of unfavourable histology treated with CHOP at initial doses reduced to 50% of the calculated full dosage [10]. Toxicity reported was generally mild, and 10 out of 11 remained continuously free of disease at the time of the report. However, 7 of the 11 patients received only 2 to 4 courses of the initial CHOP because of prolonged myelosuppression, and then were treated with radiation therapy. It is conceivable from this experience that patients who are likely to need more prolonged treatment, i.e., those with unfavourable stage III and IV disease, may not be able to receive CHOP, even at reduced doses, without significant toxicity.

More recently, Dixon et al. retrospectively analysed two SWOG studies dealing with patients with DHL and concluded that: 1) elderly (≥ 65 years) and younger adult patients with DHL present with the same clinical characteristics; 2) they obtain a similar CR rate when treated with a comparable dose of chemotherapy; and 3) there is no correlation between age and toxic side effects from CHOP [38]. The group studied by Dixon and colleagues was composed of a highly selected population of elderly patients, which had been included in the SWOG studies probably for some "favourable" clinical characteristics at diagnosis, i.e., good performance status and age less than 70. It is, indeed, surprising that Dixon et al. did not report the median age of this group of elderly patients. In fact, it is obvious that it makes a great difference, for example, whether the population they were dealing with had a median age of 67 or 75 years [39].

The results of the various groups in this Intercity Meeting were again controversial: according to the German groups, in unfavourable lymphomas of elderly people, as well as in those of the younger population, incidence, grading of toxicity and results of treatment were equivalent to those observed in cases under 70. On the other hand, in the retrospective study of the EORTC Lymphoma Group, aggressive treatment was more toxic, providing results equivalent to those of an average younger population. This study suggested that evaluation of toxic deaths in elderly patients undergoing chemotherapy could be more difficult than in younger patients, in that effects from the progression of tumour and side effects from chemotherapy are often similar and hardly distinguishable. Other data presented by the Italian group indicated that results equivalent to those obtained with standard combination chemotherapy (CHOP) can be reproduced with protocols specifically devised for elderly people (epipodophyllotoxins ± prednimustine) with less toxicity.

The explanation for these differences should probably be ascribed to patient selection: elderly patients who are in good general conditions (normal hepatic, cardiac and renal function and high performance status) can tolerate standard intensive combination chemotherapy. But it is well known that after 70 years only a minority of patients are usually judged clinically eligible for clinical trials [2]. Such a sample, as a result of this "natural selection", cannot, however, be considered representative of the general elderly population. The majority of the evaluations presented at this meeting were retrospective, therefore, eligibility criteria were not clearly stated at the beginning of treatment and were based on the evaluation of the individual physician in charge of the patient. The lack of controlled studies may, therefore, very well explain the conflicting results observed before and during this meeting. There was, however, general agreement that age may be a risk factor for inadequate treatment [40]. The population of elderly patients is more likely, on average, to have alterations in kidney and liver function, lower performance status and comorbidity, but the decision regarding the intensity of the treatment should be based on the individual risk of that particular patient. In other words, it is important that the treatment decision be based on the characteristics and conditions of the individual patient, not on characteristics thought to be associated with age. But, assuming that in a certain number of patients physiological age is less than chronological age and that they can be treated with the same treatment and dose intensity as younger patients, the problem would remain open for patients in whom aging has been producing functional impairment. In these patients, protocols devised for young patients could not simply be applied without risks. The problem is further complicated by the fact that, on the basis of biological parameters available today, it is not easy to predict which elderly patients will tolerate an intensive treatment. This can be attributed mainly to the fact that very little information is available on the pharmacokinetics of most antitumour drugs in elderly people. This information would help in constructing a model to serve as a guide to the administration of a specifically devised cancer chemotherapy for elderly patients with NHL, taking into account that in this setting, the major aim would be to prolong survival with a good quality of life.

In conclusion, prospective clinical trials are needed to define the optimal treatment of elderly patients with NHL. The study of the pharmacokinetics of anticancer drugs in elderly patients will probably, on the one hand, help to identify those patients who can tolerate intensive treatment and, on the other, provide better information for dose scheduling and new protocol design in patients with impaired organ function.

REFERENCES

1 National Cancer Institute sponsored study of classifications of non-Hodgkin's lymphomas. Summary and description of a Working Formulation for clinical use. The non-Hodgkin's lymphoma pathologic classification project. Cancer 1982 (49):2112

2 Hunter CP, Frelick RW, Feldman AR, Bavier AR, Dunlap WH, Ford L, Henson D, Macfarlane D, Smart CR, Yancik R, Yates JW: Selection factors in clinical trials: results from the community clinical oncology program physician's patient log. Cancer Treat Rep 1987 (71):559

3 Jones SE, Fuks Z, Bull M, Kadin ME, Dorfman RF, Kaplan HS, Rosenberg SA, Kin H: Non-Hodgkin's lymphomas IV. Clinicopathologic correlation in 405 cases. Cancer 1973 (31):806

4 Patchefsky AS, Brodovsky HS, Menduke H, Southard M, Brooks J, Nicklas D, Hoch WS: Non-Hodgkin's lymphomas: a clinicopathologic study of 293 cases. Cancer 1974 (34):1173

5 Nathwani BN, Kim H, Rappaport H, Solomon J, Fox M: Non-Hodgkin's lymphomas: A clinicopathologic study comparing two classifications. Cancer 1978 (41):303

6 Anderson T, Chabner BA, Young RC, Berard CW, Garvin AJ, Simon RM, DeVita VT: Malignant lymphoma I. The histology and staging of 473 patients at the National Cancer Institute. Cancer 1982 (50):2699

7 Mead GM, Macbeth FR, Williams CJ, Ryall RD, Wright DH, Whitehouse JM: Poor prognosis non-Hodgkin's lymphoma in the elderly: clinical presentation and management. Quart J Med 1984 (53):381

8 Carbone A, Tirelli U, Volpe R, Zagonel V, Manconi R, Menin A, Trovò M, Grigoletto E: Non-Hodgkin's lymphoma in the elderly. A retrospective clinicopathologic study of 50 patients. Cancer 1986 (57):2185

9 Hoerni B, Sotto JJ, Eghbali H, Sotto MF, Hoerni-Simon G, Pegourie B: Non-Hodgkin's malignant lymphomas after 80 years. 70 cases. Third International Conference on Malignant Lymphomas, Lugano, June 10-13 1987. # P9, 103

10 Miller TP, Jones SE: Initial chemotherapy for clinically localized lymphomas of unfavourable histology. Blood 1983 (62):413

11 Otter R, Gerrits WB, Kluin-Nelemans JC, Kluin PM, Stijnen T, on behalf of the Working Party NHL. Third International Conference on Malignant Lymphomas, Lugano, June 10-13 1987, # T61,128

12 Eade NR, MacLeod SM, Renton KW: Inhibition of hepatic microsomal drug metabolism by hydrazines. Can J PHysiol Pharmacol 1972 (50):721

13 Shiba DA and Weinkam B: Quantitative analysis of procarbazine, procarbazine metabolites and chemical degradation products with application to pharmacokinetic studies. J Chromatogr 1982 (229):397

14 DeVita V, Hahn M, Oliverio V: Monoamine oxidase inhibition by a new carcinostatic agent, procarbazine. Proc Soc Exp Biol Med 1965 (120):561

15 Goldstein S: The biology of aging. N Engl J Med 1971 (285):1120

16 Blum RH, Carter SK, Agre K: A clinical review of bleomycin. A new antineoplastic agent. Cancer 1973 (31):903

17 Davies DF and Shock NW: Age changes in geomerular filtration rate, effective renal plasma flow and tabula excretory capacity in adult males. J Clin Invest 1950 (29):496

18 Hansen HH, Selawry OS, Holland JF, McCall CB: The variability of individual tolerance to methotrexate in cancer patients. Br J Cancer 1971 (25):298

19 Begg CB and Carbone PP: Clinical trials and drug toxicity in the elderly. Cancer 1983 (52):1986

20 Kuse R, Calavrezos A, Stellbrink HJ, Hielmann HP: Langzeiterfolge bei 172 hochmalignen Nicht-Hodgkin-Lymphome unter besonderer Berücksichtigung älterer Patienten. Dtsch med Wschr 1987 (112):335

21 Crom WR, Glynn-Barnhart AM, Rodman JH, Teresi ME, Kavanagh RE, Christensen ML, Relling MV, Evans WE: Pharmacokinetics of anticancer drugs in children. Clin Pharmacokinet 1987 (12):168

22 Powis G: Effects of disease states on pharmacokinetics of anticancer drugs. In: Ames MM, Powis G, Kovcach JS (eds) Pharmacokinetics of anticancer agents in humans. Elsevier, Amsterdam 1983 p 363

23 Kerr IG, Jolivet J, Collins JM, Drake JC, Chabner BA: Test dose for predicting high-dose methotrexate infusion. Clin Pharmacol Ther 1983 (33):444

24 Monjanel S, Rigault JP, Cano JP, Carcassone Y, Favre R: High-dose methotrexate. Preliminary evaluation of pharmacokinetic approach. Cancer Chemother Pharmacol 1979 (3):189

25 Bagley V, Bostick FW, DeVita VT: Clinical pharmacology of cyclophosphamide. Cancer Res 1973 (33):226

26 Bramwell V, Calvert RT, Edwards G, Scarffe H, Crowther D: The disposition of cyclophosphamide in a group of myeloma patients. Cancer Chemother Pharmacol 1979 (3):253

27 Loo TL, Hansholder GE, Gerulath AH, Saunders PH, Farquhar D: Mechanism of action and pharmacologic studies DTIC (NSC-45388). Cancer Treat Rep 1976 (60):149

28 Clark PI and Slevin ML: The clinical pharmacology of etoposide and teniposide. Clin Pharmacokinet 1987 (12):223

29 Benjamin RS: A practical approach to adriamycin (NSC 123127). Cancer Chemother Rep 1975 (6):191

30 Robert J and Hoerni B: Age dependence of the early-phase pharmacokinetics of doxorubicin. Cancer Res 1983 (43):4467

31 Bender RA and Chabner BA: Tubulin binding agents. In: Chabner BA (ed) Pharmacologic Principles of Cancer Treatment. WB Saunders Co, Philadelphia 1982 p 229

32 Brittinger G, Bartels H, Common H, Duhmke E, Fulle HH, Gunzer U, Gyenes T, Heinz R, Konig E, Meusers P: Clinical and prognostic relevance of the Kiel classification of non-Hodgkin's lymphomas. Results of a prospective multicenter study by the

Kiel Lymphoma Study Group. Haematol Oncol 1984 (2):269
33 Zagonel V, Tirelli U, Veronesi A et al: Non-Hodgkin's lymphomas in the elderly: increase in lethal and severe toxicity without improvement in survival with aggressive therapy vs conservative therapy. Proc International Symposium on Recent Approaches to Chronic Lymphoproliferative Disease. Prague, September 1975
34 Armitage JO, Potter JF: Aggressive chemotherapy for diffuse histiocytic lymphoma in the elderly: increased complications with advancing age. J Am Geriatr Soc 1984 (32):269
35 Tirelli U, Carbone A, Crivellari D, Volpe R, Franchin G, Veronesi A, Galligioni E, Trovò M, Tumolo S, Grigoletto E: A phase II trial of Teniposide (VM26) in advanced non-Hodgkin's lymphoma, with emphasis on the treatment of the elderly patients. Cancer 1984 (54):393
36 Tirelli U, Carbone A, Zagonel V, Veronesi A, Canetta R: Non-Hodgkin's lymphomas in the elderly: prospective studies with specifically devised chemotherapy regimens in 66 patients. Eur J Cancer Clin Oncol 1987 (23):535
37 Tirelli U on behalf of the EORTC Lymphoma Group: Treatment-related toxicity in elderly patients with malignant lymphoma (letter). J Clin Oncol 1987 (5):679
38 Dixon DO, Neilan B, Jones SE, Lipschitz DA, Miller TP, Grozea PN, Wilson HE: Effects of age and therapeutic outcome in advanced diffuse histiocytic lymphoma: the Southwest Oncology Group experience. J Clin Oncol 1986 (4):295
39 Zagonel V, Tirelli U, Carbone A: Treatment of non-Hodgkin's lymphoma in the elderly (letter). J Clin Oncol 1986 (12):1866
40 Wetle T: Age as a risk factor for inadequate treatment. JAMA 1987 (258):516

Management of Non-Hodgkin's Lymphomas: Conclusions of the Third Intercity Meeting, 1988

J. Estapé [1], L. Brandao [2], N. de Lena [3], J. Garcia-Conde [4], J. Gary Bobo [5], J.A. Gastaut [6], P. Mazza [7] and E. Montserrat [8]

1 Oncology Service, Hospital Clinic, Barcelona, Spain
2 Institute of Oncology, Coimbra, Portugal
3 Ospedale Oncologico, Bari, Italy
4 Haemato-oncology Service, Hospital Clinico, Valencia, Spain
5 Centre Paul Lamarque, Montpellier, France
6 Haematology Service, Institut J. Paoli - I. Calmettes, Marseille, France
7 Haematology Institute S. and A. Seragnoli, Bologna, Italy
8 School of Haematology, Hospital Clinic, Barcelona, Spain

A third Intercity Meeting under the auspices of the European School of Oncology was held in Barcelona on 27th May, 1988. The subject of the meeting was the current management of non-Hodgkin's lymphoma (NHL) and the results of the discussion are reported in this paper.

Low-Grade NHL

It was found that on the rare occasions (10-20%) when patients present with limited (stages I and II), low-grade NHL, and are treated with involved or extended field radiotherapy with or without chemotherapy, results prove to be very similar, however, when combined therapy is administered, disease-free survival (DFS) is longer [1,2]. The great majority of patients present with advanced disease (stages III and IV) and, in the presence of indolent diffuse lymphocytic, well-differentiated lymphoma with no risk factors, it was reported that therapy could be withheld until such time as the progress of the disease made it mandatory. Such an approach does not compromise the final outcome for the patient [3]. For those cases in which treatment is used, a single alkylating agent, or a combination therapy can be given. Combination therapy is considered more appropriate when there is a need for the tumour burden to be reduced rapidly [4,5]. However, since this "watch and wait" strategy has no effect on survival, several trials have been initiated comparing this abstention strategy with treatment started on diagnosis. Young et al. [6] have reported some very interesting results: they randomly compared the "watch and wait" strategy with ProMACE-MOPP (followed by total nodal irradiation), and found that both approaches gave similar survival rates, though the aggressive approach provided statistically significant DFS rates. According to Young et al. [6], initial aggressive therapy is the only means for patients to be maintained continuously disease free. This experience, together with other similar trials, could be a starting point for modifying the natural history of low grade NHLs. On the other hand, patients presenting with risk factors on diagnosis must be treated early. Prognostic factors, such as B symptoms, hepatosplenomegaly, anaemia and abnormal liver function, correlated with short survival [8].

Intermediate-Grade and Immunoblastic Type

With intermediate grade of malignancy and the immunoblastic type, treatment has to be more aggressive and authors agree that bone marrow transplantation is being more frequently used throughout. The rate of complete response (CR) ranges from 39% to 83% with chemotherapy alone, bearing in mind the wide variation of prognostic factors (bulky disease, bone marrow involvement), histological subtypes and other selection criteria [7]. It has been shown that an increasing number of institutions are making use of third-generation regimens, such as induction chemotherapy and others, thereby improving the CR rate and, in all probability, survival also. However, in order to identify the true contribution of aggressive versus standard chemotherapy regimens in these patients, several trials were set up [9]. The Spanish Cooperative Group (PETHEMA) implemented a randomised trial comparing CHOP to ProMACE-CytaBOM in intermediate grade and immunoblastic NHL, stages II and IV [10]. Up to the present time, 104 patients have been accrued (87 now evaluable). Overall CR rates are 59% and 61%, respectively. No differences were observed either in median survival probability (MSP), or in DFS probability. Toxicity was higher in the ProMACE-CytaBOM arm. Low-risk patients showed a significantly higher MSP than high-risk patients. The serum lactic dehydrogenase (LDH) level of less than 450 UI/l is the main single positive prognostic factor. According to several preliminary reports [9,10], results measured in a cooperative group show no difference between the two schedules. The CR rate is similar throughout the groups, but a major problem to be clarified is whether DFS will improve with an aggressive regimen.

Some discussion was also dedicated to the role of chemotherapy, or radiotherapy, or a combination of both techniques, with bone marrow transplantation as a consolidation therapy. As was shown previously [11,12], autologous bone marrow transplantation (ABMT) performed for bulky or refractory disease is less effective than ABMT in second or first CR. As a demonstration of this technique, the results of a trial carried out at the Institut J. Paoli - I. Calmettes (Marseilles) were presented. Seventy-two NHL patients were treated with several induction regimens; most of them (46%) were engrafted in first CR, 16 (22%) in second CR, or later (CR ≥ 2 years) and 23 (32%) in relapse. Twenty-one patients (29%) had intermediate-grade NHL and 10 (14%) immunoblastic NHL. Initial status (first or second CR or relapse) correlated well with survival, showing in multivariate analysis that status is highly significant ($p < 0.006$). In accordance with these data, BMT for NHL is of no advantage in relapsing patients. This trial showed that BMT is more or less equivalent to ABMT, since they are conditioning regimens with or without total body irradiation, in the same way as bone marrow purging may be. Pilot studies analysing BMT prospectively in first CR have already shown some encouraging results in poor-risk intermediate grade NHL, as well as in immunoblastic NHL. Maintenance of prolonged DFS (and possible cure) justifies consolidation treatment with massive therapy and early BMT in poor-risk NHL. One point that has to be more clearly defined is the identification of true prognostic factors to justify early BMT.

Lymphoblastic and Burkitt's Lymphomas

Among diffuse, aggressive malignant lymphomas, lymphoblastic (LBL) and Burkitt's lymphoma (BL) are two different entities. They are differentiated by their origin, LBL originating from the T-cell, while BL from the B-cell. Incidence of these two NHLs being low, clinical research proves to be rather difficult. Conventional therapy of these lymphomas has also yielded dismal results, however, newer therapeutic protocols, using intensified chemotherapy programmes with induction, consolidation, maintenance and central nervous system (CNS) prophylaxis, have led to a remarkable improvement in the overall prognosis of both diseases.

With regard to lymphoblastic lymphoma, Anderson et al. [13] demonstrated the superiority of employing large numbers of drugs versus the conventional treatment of lymphomas. Duque Hammershaimb et al. [14] confirmed this same tendency in young patients, with 64% DFS at 4 years of age. A recent review by Slater [15] stressed the prognostic factors in LBL: over 30 years of age, WBC more than 50,000/ml, failure to achieve CR and late CR during induction were indicators of poor prognosis. On the other hand, peripheral blood involvement at presentation, T-cell surface markers and the presence of a mediastinal mass did not adversely affect survival. The following preliminary conclusions can, therefore, be drawn: in the treatment of LBL, 1) multidrug regimens, particularly those which include induction therapy, consolidation and maintenance chemotherapy are more effective than conventional 3-4 drug regimens; 2) early prophylaxis of CNS relapse with both irradiation and i.t. MTX can really reduce relapses at this site; 3) high-risk patients should receive more intensive chemotherapy programmes; 4) mediastinal radiotherapy is not useful, unless it is used for symptomatic relief of superior vena cava syndromes, which frequently occur in these patients. The duration of the treatment and the best treatment programme to adopt still have to be defined.

A further point to be investigated in more detail is the treatment of patients who do not achieve CR, or those who relapse on therapy. The treatment of choice might be bone marrow transplantation for these patients, but long-term results are still disappointing [16]; whereas, high-risk patients might benefit from this treatment during first complete remission, as was suggested by Nademanee [17].

In the discussion on Burkitt's lymphoma, it was pointed out that first-line treatment should be a surgical reduction of the bulk of the tumour, due to the strict relationship between the volume of the tumour and prognosis [18]. Then metabolic stability must be achieved early - control of serum levels in particular - and, following an as complete and rapid staging as possible, adequate chemotherapy must be initiated. Several chemotherapeutic agents are active in BL.

In recent years, a significant improvement of overall survival has been seen in African and American patients [19] treated with combination chemotherapy, combined modality treatment and prevention of CNS involvement. The most important progress found with combination chemotherapy was the dramatic improvement in the relapse rate. Several regimens were evaluated; BL and other undifferentiated rapidly growing lymphomas are potentially curable diseases under the following conditions: 1) diagnosis should be established within a maximum of 48 hours. In order to initiate therapy as quickly as possible, staging should be limited to CT scans of the abdomen and the thorax, ultrasound examination of the abdomen, lumbar puncture and bone marrow aspiration; 2) bulky tumour, if easily accessible, should be removed to reduce the tumour burden (particularly in young patients); 3) multiagent chemotherapy should be given as soon as possible; 4) to prevent or to treat metabolic abnormalities, it is mandatory to treat patients with allopurinol, hydration with alkalinisation, or haemodialysis if necessary; 5) radiotherapy is usually unnecessary, but should be considered if there is incomplete tumour regression following chemotherapy; 6) CNS prophylaxis is mandatory; chemotherapy alone is probably inadequate; 7) new therapeutic approaches are needed for poor-risk patients, because of the high percentage of relapses still occurring. More intensive chemotherapy should be considered for these patients, with or without bone marrow transplantation.

Salvage Treatment

The prognosis of patients with recurrent or refractory NHL is known to be extremely poor, especially in cases of aggressive types of lymphoma [20]. Several schedules of salvage chemotherapy have been reported, but up to now none of them were reported as acceptable and satisfactory worldwide. The work concerning salvage chemotherapy in NHL to which one can refer is that by Cabanillas et al. [21].

Resistance to first-line therapy could be defined as the persistence of the disease on termination of treatment and could be classified into two distinct categories of patients: those who do not respond to therapy, or in whom the disease continues to progress whilst in therapy, and those who have a partial response. Relapse was defined as a recurrence of symptoms, or other signs indicating lymphoma. An analysis is reported here of a study conducted on a population of 646 unselected patients observed at the Institute of Haematology "L. and A. Seragnoli", Bologna, between 1970 and 1985. All histologies under the Kiel classification were represented

[22]. Staging procedures were those conventionally established at the Ann Arbor Conference. Due to the length of the accrual period, both the induction therapy and that of the resistant or relapsing patients were quite variable (CVP, MEV or CHOP, BACOP, MEVAP in high-grade NHL patients). After 1982, high-risk NHL patients received more intensive treatment: a modification of the LSA_2-L_2 regimen for patients with bone marrow involvement or over 40 years of age; massive chemotherapy followed by autologous bone marrow transplantation [23] for patients without bone marrow involvement and under 45 years of age. In resistant or relapsing patients the therapy was variable also, in accordance with the previous schedule and the protocol used at the time of resistance or relapse. A significant difference in survival was recorded among patients who were either primarily resistant, partially responding, or who relapsed to first-line therapy. Efforts should be directed in particular at patients who obtained some response, or who relapsed following first-line chemotherapy and not at those who are truly resistant. We can suppose that a lymphoma which proves to be truly resistant to a scheme that is widely considered to be effective as a first-line therapy, will rarely have a stable response to a second-line therapy.
Progress in salvage treatment of NHL is important, but at present there are no satisfactory treatments available. However, despite the fact that the results are not exciting, only 20% of patients surviving at 2 years [21], this approach provided a few leads for future trends in resistant or relapsed NHL: 1) alternative schemes for first-line therapy should include new drugs which are not cross-resistant with those used previously; 2) therapeutic efforts should be particularly directed towards patients who obtained some response, or who relapsed after first-line chemotherapy; 3) therapy should be intensified, involving ABMT or allogeneic bone marrow transplantation. Nevertheless, in those patients who are truly resistant, no more than 10% can be salvaged by these procedures [23]. In the other patients, a 40% longer survival was observed [24], with the possibility of a cure for most of them. Unfortunately, the majority of these patients are not eligible for such procedures, due to age factors, bone marrow involvement or the absence of a compatible donor.

Conclusions

In conclusion, we found that:

1) in limited disease (stages I and II), low- and intermediate-grade NHL, the treatment of choice will be radiotherapy, with or without chemotherapy;
2) in advanced quiescent low-grade NHL, it seemed until now mandatory to withhold therapy, but a more aggressive initial therapy could improve disease-free survival and change its natural history;
3) in stages II and IV, intermediate and immunoblastic NHL, the CHOP regimen is the standard chemotherapy to compare with more aggressive schedules. Bone marrow transplantation as a consolidation therapy could increase survival following chemotherapy, since the results are better in those patients engrafted in first complete remission;
4) progress in the treatment of high-grade NHL has been impressive in the last 20 years. Lymphoblastic lymphoma is a potentially curable disease, even though further studies are needed to improve the prognosis of high-risk patients. Burkitt's lymphoma is also a potentially curable disease, but management of this disease requires special attention. For both these diseases at a refractory stage, clinical research on bone marrow transplantation is in progress;
5) progress in salvage treatment for NHL with aggressive chemotherapy is significant, though no satisfactory treatment is at present available. The inclusion of new non-cross-resistant drugs in first-line therapy and the intensification of treatment, with the probable inclusion of BMT, could be the future trend in the management of this disease.

REFERENCES

1 Portlock CS: "Good risk" non-Hodgkin's lymphomas: approaches to management. Sem Hematol 1983 (20):25-34
2 Kinsella TJ: Role of combined-modality therapy in the curative management of advanced-stage "favorable" non-Hodgkin's lymphomas. Cancer Treat Rep 1982 (66):421-426
3 Montserrat E, Gardella S, Llebaria C, Rozman C: Deferral of initial therapy in advanced "favorable" lymphomas. In: Sotto JJ et al (eds) Non-Hodgkin's Lymphomas: New Techniques and Treatments. Karger, Basle 1985 pp 215-220
4 De Vita VT Jr, Longo DL, Hubbard SM, Young RC, Chabner BA: The lymphomas: biologic implications of therapy and therapeutic implications of the new biology. In: Malignant Lymphoma. Williams & Wilkins, Baltimore 1987 pp 249-267
5 Giralt M, Montserrat E, Maldonado J et al: Terapéutica de los limfomas no hodgkinianos clínicamente agresivos en estadios III y IV con CHOP. Neoplasia 1986 (3):119-124
6 Young RC, Longo DL, Glatstein E, Ihde DC, Jaffe ES and De Vita VT Jr: The treatment of indolent lymphomas: watchful and waiting vs aggressive combined modality treatment. Sem Hematol Vol 25, No 2, suppl 2 1988 pp 11-16
7 Lee R, Cabanillas F, Bodey GP, Freireich EJ: A 10-year update of CHOP-Bleo in the treatment of diffuse large-cell lymphoma. J Clin Oncol 1986 (4):1455-1461
8 McLaughlin P, Fuller LM, Velasquez WS et al: Stage III follicular lymphoma: durable remissions with a combined chemotherapy-radiotherapy regimen. J Clin Oncol 1987 (5):867-874
9 Miller ThP, Dana BW, Weick JK et al: Southwest Oncology Group Clinical Trials for intermediate and high grade non-Hodgkin's lymphomas. Sem Hematol Vol 25 No 2 suppl 2 pp 1988 17-22
10 Programa para el estudio y el tratamiento de las hemopatias malignas (PETHEMA). Protocolo XXI, linfomas no Hodgkin, CHOP-ProMACE CytaBOM
11 Philip T, Armitage JO, Spitzer G et al: High-dose therapy and autologous bone marrow transplantation after failure of conventional chemotherapy in adults with intermediate-grade or high-grade non-Hodgkin's lymphoma. N Engl J Med 1987 (316):1493-1498
12 Takvorian T, Canellos GP, Ritz J et al: Prolonged disease-free survival after autologous bone marrow transplantation in patients with non-Hodgkin's lymphoma with a poor prognosis. N Engl J Med 1987 (316):1499-1505
13 Anderson JR, Wilson JF, Jenkin DT et al: Childhood non-Hodgkin's lymphomas: results of a randomized therapeutic trial comparing a 4-drug regimen (COMP) to a 10-drug regimen (LSA2 L2). N Engl J Med 1983 (308):559
14 Duque-Hammershaimb L, Wollner N, Miller DR: LSA2-L2 protocol treatment of stage IV non-Hodgkin's lymphoma in children with partial and extensive bone marrow involvement. Cancer 1983 (52):39
15 Slater DE, Mertelsmann R, Koziner B et al: Lymphoblastic lymphoma in adults. J Clin Oncol 1986 (4):57
16 Philip T, Armitage JO, Spitzer G et al: High dose therapy and autologous bone marrow transplantation after failure of conventional chemotherapy in adults with intermediate grade or high grade non-Hodgkin's lymphoma. New Engl J Med 1987 (316):1493
17 Nademanee AP, Foreman JJ, Schmidt GM et al: Allogenic bone marrow transplantation for high risk non-Hodgkin's lymphoma during first complete remission. Blut 1987 (55):11
18 Magrath I, Lee YJ, Anderson T et al: Prognostic factors in Burkitt's lymphoma: importance of total tumor burden. Cancer 1980 (45):1507
19 Ziegler JL: Burkitt's lymphoma. New Engl J Med 1981 (305):735
20 Coiffier B, Bosly A, Galligaris-Cappio F et al, European School of Oncology: Management of non-Hodgkin's lymphomas: conclusions of the European School of Oncology meeting, 1986. Eur J Cancer Clin Oncol 1987 (23):1691-1695
21 Cabanillas F, Hagemeister FB, Riggs S et al: Results of iphosphamide-etoposide combinations for patients with recurrent or refractory aggressive lymphoma. In: Cavalli F, Bonadonna G, Rozencweig M (eds) Malignant Lymphomas and Hodgkin's Disease: Experimental and Therapeutic Advances. 1985 p 485
22 Lennert T, Mohori M, Stein H: The histopathology of malignant lymphoma. Br J Haematol 1975 (31 suppl):193-203
23 Zinzani PL, Gherlinzoni F, Lauria F et al: Intensive chemotherapy regimen in high-grade non-Hodgkin's lymphomas. Tumori 1987 (73):121-126
24 Tura S, Mazza P, Gherlinzoni F et al: High-dose therapy followed by autologous bone marrow transplantation (ABMT) in previously untreated non-Hodgkin's lymphomas. Scand J Haematol 1986 (37):347-352

Management of Non-Hodgkin's Lymphomas in Adults in Scandinavia, the United Kingdom and the Netherlands: Conclusions of the Fourth Intercity Meeting, 1988

Gunnar Juliusson [1], Arne F. Abrahamsen [4], Eva Cavallin-Ståhl [3], Anthony H. Goldstone[6], Andrew Lister [7], Nis I. Nissen [5], Karl-Hendrik Robèrt [1], Charles R.J. Singer [6], Reinier Somers [8], Åke Öst [2] and Gösta Gahrton [1]

1 Division of Clinical Haematology and Oncology, Department of Medicine, Karolinska Institute at Huddinge Hospital, Huddinge, Sweden
2 Department of Pathology, Karolinska Hospital, Stockholm, Sweden
3 Department of Oncology, University Hospital, Lund, Sweden
4 Department of Medical Oncology, The Norwegian Radium Hospital, Oslo, Norway
5 Department of Haematology, The Finsen Institute, Copenhagen, Denmark
6 Department of Haematology, University College Hospital, London, United Kingdom
7 Department of Medical Oncology, St. Bartholomew's Hospital, London, United Kingdom
8 Department of Medicine, The Netherlands Cancer Institute, Amsterdam, The Netherlands

The fourth Intercity Meeting of the European School of Oncology on non-Hodgkin's lymphoma, chaired by Professor Gösta Gahrton, was held at Huddinge Hospital on 3rd June, 1988. The purpose of the meeting was to present and challenge current treatment strategies in Scandinavia, the United Kingdom and the Netherlands. The discussion was based on the following papers: "Critical analysis of pretreatment staging in non-Hodgkin's lymphoma" (Öst), "High-grade malignant non-Hodgkin's lymphoma in Norway. Treatment and clinical aspects" (Abrahamsen), "EORTC studies in malignant lymphoma" (Somers), "Management of high-grade malignant non-Hodgkin's lymphoma. Report from a Swedish multi-centre study" (Cavallin-Ståhl), "Biological tumour progression in low-grade malignant non-Hodgkin's lymphoma" (Nissen), "Management of follicular lymphoma" (Lister), and "Bone marrow transplantation in non-Hodgkin's lymphoma" (Goldstone).

Reprinted with permission from Reviews in Oncology 2 (1989) 1 (in Acta Oncologica Vol. 28, Fasc. 1, pp 135-140)

Tumour Progression

The general concept of a tumour is that of a dynamic population of cells in which there is a gradual acquisition of new characteristics as the tumour develops. A genetic instability of the tumour is the basis for a high mutation rate with formation of new subclones leading to tumour heterogeneity. Thus, a subsequent overgrowth of one or more new subclones can thus lead to a more aggressive clinical picture and to resistance to treatment.

This multistep progression is classically seen in follicular small cleaved cell lymphoma and in chronic myelocytic leukaemia (CML). Both these diseases are characterised by an initial indolent phase, easy to control by a non-aggressive treatment. Cytogenetic markers, t(14;18) and t(9;22) (i.e., the Philadelphia chromosome), respectively, are present in almost all cases. In a non-predictable way both diseases may progress to a clinically more aggressive disease characterised by 1) conversion of morphology to large-cell lymphoma with diffuse histological pattern [1] and blastic crisis, respectively; 2) additional chromosome abnormalities, such as del(13), del(6), or +12 [2] in follicular lymphoma, and another Ph chromosome, +8, or iso(17q) in CML [3,4]; 3) new tumour cell characteristics with invasion and metastasis to areas usually not involved in the chronic phase; 4) increased tumour cell proliferation rate; 5) increased tumour cell resistance to cytostatic treatment and 6) short survival of only a few months after conversion. The conversion is not induced by chemotherapy. Histological conversion is often found in biopsies from relapses at new and atypical sites.

This finding in follicular lymphoma and CML contrasts to that of chronic lymphocytic leukaemia (CLL), in which clinical progression usually is not accompanied by changes in the CLL-cell phenotype, cytology or chromosome patterns [5].

The clonogenic tumour is not the granulocyte in CML, nor the small cleaved cell of follicular lymphoma. In follicular lymphoma the typical chromosomal translocation, with the juxtapositioning of the *bcl*-2 oncogene from chromosome 18 to the VJ region of the immunoglobulin heavy chain locus of chromosome 14 [6], is indicative of a malignant transformation of an early pre-B cell, in which the immunoglobulin gene rearrangements normally take place. The clonogenic cells of these malignancies can be described as primitive tumour cells with the ability to differentiate, but during the gradual progression this ability is lost.

Pretreatment Staging in Non-Hodgkin's Lymphoma

Classification

The pretreatment staging consists of two parts - both essential to the management of the individual patient. The first part is the analysis of the lymphoma cells and their growth patterns, most importantly performed by morphology and immune phenotyping, and the second part is the localisation and spread of the disease, detected by physical examination, radiological methods and morphology/cytology.

The Kiel classification (for the revised nomenclature, see ref. 7) is mostly used in Scandinavia. The EORTC has suggested a slightly different grouping, which emphasises the prognostic importance of the tumour cell growth pattern: 1) a low-grade malignant group consisting of low-grade Kiel types with follicular growth pattern (80% 5-year survival); 2) an intermediate group with low-grade Kiel types with diffuse growth (50% 5-year survival) and 3) a high-grade malignant group with high-grade Kiel types with diffuse growth pattern (35% 5-year survival) [8].

Staging

The Ann Arbor staging system was developed for Hodgkin's disease but has been adopted and generally used in non-Hodgkin's lymphomas, although most studies do not show prognostic differences between stages II, III and IV. However, no better staging system is available. The important matters are agreed to be 1) that stage I patients should have a meticulous investigation, and 2) that patients with stage II-IV disease should receive systemic treatment.

Histology and immune phenotyping must be performed on tissue from the major site of the lymphoma, whereas if there is doubt about involvement in other regions, fine-needle aspiration with immune phenotyping could be sufficient. It is generally assumed that in lymphoma patients enlarged lymph nodes are involved with lymphoma, whereas those with normal size are not. However, this assumption is not supported by specific studies.

Sites of Involvement

Abdomen. Different radiological methods were discussed. In some centres computerised tomography has replaced lymphangiography as the routine method for analysis of abdominal and retroperitoneal lymph nodes, although the latter method has the advantage that the lymph node structure can be studied and also has a greater sensitivity in the lower peritoneum. Thus, lymphangiography was recommended in stage I patients with a normal abdominal computerised tomography.

Chest. Of all lymphoma patients about 40% have shown to have intrathoracic involvement

[9]. Regarding mediastinal lymph nodes and lung parenchymal involvement, computerised tomography and magnetic resonance imaging are more sensitive than routine radiography, but if the latter is abnormal no valuable information will be added by the other radiological methods [10]. Pleural involvement is usually accompanied by effusion, which allows cytology and immune phenotyping.

Bone marrow. Bone marrow involvement was frequently found in low-grade malignant lymphomas (77%) and lymphoblastic lymphomas (39%), but is less frequent in other high-grade malignant lymphomas (24%) and centroblastic/centrocytic lymphomas (20%) [11]. False-negative aspirations are especially common in immunocytomas and follicle-centre cell derived lymphomas where fibrosis may occur. A bone biopsy should always be performed if the marrow aspiration is negative.

Blood. A clonal B-cell excess in the peripheral blood (normal blood lymphocyte count but a k/l ratio outside the normal range 1.0-3.3) can be found in B-cell lymphomas even without bone marrow involvement [12]. This analysis is not routinely performed but was advocated.

Spleen. Enlarged spleens of lymphoma patients should be regarded as involved with lymphoma [13], but so are one-third of normal-sized spleens. Fine-needle aspiration with immune phenotyping should be performed to exclude splenic involvement in patients who are considered for local therapy only. Excision biopsy was not recommended because of the high risk of complications [14].

Liver. The liver is involved in 15% of lymphoma patients [13]. Radionucleid scans have greater sensitivity and specificity than computerised tomography. Liver, but not bone marrow involvement was in an EORTC study found to be an adverse prognostic factor. It was discussed whether liver biopsy should be performed in all patients, but the small chance of getting a positive biopsy in patients without clinical signs of liver involvement does not justify the risk.

Gastrointestinal tract. Half of all gastrointestinal lymphomas are localised to the stomach, one-third to the small intestine, and one-eighth to the ileocaecal region, whereas other sites are uncommon [15]. Barium investigation and endoscopy should be performed when involvement is suspected. Endoscopic ultrasonography yields a high specificity [16].

Central nervous system. Involvement of the central nervous system is fairly common in lymphoblastic lymphomas (23%) [17], and cytology of cerebrospinal fluid with immune phenotyping is recommended as an initial routine in high-grade lymphomas and always if symptoms from the central nervous system occur.

Bone. Primary bone lymphomas comprise one-fourth of extranodal lymphomas and constitute 1% of primary bone tumours [18]. One-fourth of lymphoma patients will get bone involvement during the course of the disease, but few have it at diagnosis. Scanning methods are to be preferred, but should be used only if symptoms are present.

Management of Low-Grade Malignant Non-Hodgkin's Lymphoma

Follicular lymphomas have, according to previous studies with 20 years of follow up, a natural course with a fairly constant death rate and a 5-year survival of 40-50% [19]. Recent programmes aim to improve survival through more aggressive interventions.

Stage I Disease

Of 147 patients studied at St. Bartholomew's Hospital in London, 11 with follicular stage I disease received radiotherapy and had a good survival. Adjuvant chemotherapy did not seem to improve the results. However, in an EORTC study on 124 patients with stage I disease, all histologies, all patients received radiotherapy to involved and adjacent lymph node regions, 2 Gy daily up to 40 Gy. They were then randomised to receive adjuvant chemotherapy, i.e., 12 courses CVP (vincristine 2 mg day 1, cyclophosphamide 300 mg/m^2 and prednisone 40 mg/m^2 orally on day 1 through 5), or a similar regimen, versus no further treatment. The chemotherapy improved the relapse-free survival (75% vs 55% at 5 years), but overall survival was 85% at 5 years in both groups [8].

Stage II-IV Disease

Asymptomatic Disease. The "watch and wait" policy in asymptomatic generalised disease is shown to give the same results as treatment from diagnosis [1]. In asymptomatic CLL with Binet stage A, survival is impaired in patients treated with chlorambucil daily from diagnosis as compared to initially untreated patients [20]. Untreated patients should also be seen in the regional centres and not by general practitioners only. It was pointed out that the asymptomatic patients ought to be the best selection of patients, and they should have a better prognosis than therapy-demanding patients and not just as good. It might be those patients who are possible to cure permanently.

Single-agent chemotherapy. At St. Bartholomew's Hospital 111 stage III and IV patients with follicular lymphoma had a linear survival curve with a median survival of 9 years and no plateau [19]. Patients received chlorambucil 10 mg daily for 6 weeks plus 3 2-week cycles. The response rate at presentation, first relapse and second relapse was 75%, with the median duration of the first, second and third remissions being the same (18 months). The median survival in second, third and fourth remission was 6, 4 and 2 years, respectively. Those who achieved a good partial remission did just as well as those who went into complete remission.

Interferon. Interferon (IFN) has been shown to be an active agent in follicular lymphoma [21], and synergy between IFN and alkylating agents has been demonstrated in nude mice with breast cancer. Therefore, several centres have performed randomised trials comparing chlorambucil and IFN with chlorambucil alone. However, the experience from an ongoing study at St. Bartholomew's Hospital showed no difference in response rate. Furthermore, the combination was associated with greater haematological toxicity than chlorambucil alone.

Combination chemotherapy. The CVP regimen did not improve survival more than chlorambucil alone, and a high-dose chemotherapy programme with cyclophosphamide (2.5 g/m^2) and prednisone was highly toxic and discontinued.

It was discussed if doxorubicin improves the results, but no randomised trial to specifically evaluate this critical issue is available. In an EORTC study the 5-year survival for follicular stage III-IV lymphoma treated with doxorubicin, teniposide, cyclophosphamide and prednisone (CICS or CHVmP) was 72%, being significantly better than for low-grade malignant lymphomas with diffuse histology (45% at 5 years), whereas the relapse-free survival was not different between the follicular and the diffuse subgroups. In another EORTC study on follicular lymphoma stage III-IV comparing CICS chemotherapy to total body irradiation (TBI, 25 times 0.1 Gy, given 3 times a week plus booster radiotherapy on areas with a slow regression of tumour), a higher complete remission rate was achieved by chemotherapy than by TBI (55% and 36%, respectively); however, total response rates, relapse-free survival and survival were not different.

A meeting report on ProMACE-MOPP (prednisone, methotrexate, doxorubicin, cyclophosphamide, etoposide, mustargen, vincristine, procarbazine) was referred to, showing promising results in folicular lymphoma with long-term freedom of recurrence [22].

The Lymphoma Group of Central Sweden runs a randomised trial between chlorambucil/prednisolone ad modum Knospe [23] versus CHOP (cyclophosphamide, doxorubicin, vincristine, prednisone) [24] for symptomatic stage II-IV low-grade malignant lymphoma, showing equal survival for the chronic lymphocytic leukaemia and immunocytoma subgroups, but a non-significant advantage for the CHOP regimen in the centroblastic/centrocytic follicular lymphomas.

Autologous bone marrow transplantation. At St. Bartholomew's Hospital 20 patients (mean age 43 years; range 29-61 years) have been treated with high-dose cyclophosphamide and TBI with ABMT in second or subsequent remission of follicular lymphoma. Most patients were stage III-IV initially, and 9 had bone marrow involvement. The bone marrow was treated *in vitro* with the monoclonal antibody anti-B1 (from Coulter Immunology) and complement. Fifteen patients are in continuous complete remission (median follow up 18 months), 2 have relapsed with blastic transformation after 10 months and 22 months, respectively, one relapsed with the same histology after 2 years, one died of fungal infection after granulocyte but not platelet recovery, and one died from another cause, in remission. These data are encouraging but, of course, preliminary.

Management of High-Grade Malignant Non-Hodgkin's Lymphoma

CHOP and CHOP-like Regimens

In Norway 118 patients with high-grade malignant lymphoma stage II-IV (mostly stage IV) were treated during the period 1981-1984. Patients with lymphoblastic lymphomas (mean age 28 years) had a poor prognosis on CHOP with CNS treatment (one of 19 surviving for more than 2 years), and are now selected for autologous bone marrow transplantation (ABMT) in first remission.

The centroblastic and immunoblastic lymphomas occurred in older patients, mean age 67 years, and most patients under 80 years of age received CHOP. The results were age-dependent: long-term survival in patients under 55 years old was 75%, and 60% in those under 60. These results are comparable with those reported from other centres using intensive multi-drug strategies. Thus, it is still not clear whether such third-generation regimens improve survival compared with the conventional CHOP treatment. Patients in Norway who entered a complete remission had an 80% long-term survival, and thus ABMT was not recommended in first complete remission in these histological subgroups but only in good partial remission and second complete remission.

The Swedish Lymphoma study collected 196 evaluable patients with high-grade malignant lymphoma stage II-IV (including also 5 patients with a bulky stage I disease) from 1983 to 1986. Median age was 65 years. Patients were randomised to receive CHOP every third week versus CHOP with additional medium-dose methotrexate (250 mg/m^2) on day 14. The complete remission rate was 56% versus 67%, but there was no difference in relapse-free survival (one-third at 3 years) or survival (38% at 3.5 years). It was found that patients receiving methotrexate more often needed dose reduction of cyclophosphamide and doxorubicin, which might explain the lack of difference in efficacy between the 2 regimens.

The dose intensity of cyclophosphamide and doxorubicin was also evaluated in the Norwegian study. Most of the long-term survivors had had the calculated dose, whereas only 35% of those who died during the first year had received ≥ 90% of the calculated dose. It was pointed out in the discussion that the ability to tolerate a full-dose regimen is a good prognostic factor.

The EORTC has performed a similar study with CICS (doxorubicin 50 mg/m^2 day 1, teniposide 60 mg/m^2 day 1, cyclophosphamide 300 mg/m^2 day 3-4, prednisone 40 mg/m^2 days 3-7) every third week with or without vincristine and bleomycin on day 15 [8]. The complete remission rate and survival were significantly greater in the arm with additional chemotherapy (73% versus 48% and 63% versus 40% at 3 years, respectively).

Third-Generation Therapy

The MACOP-B (methotrexate, doxorubicin, cyclophosphamide, vincristine, prednisone, bleomycin) regimen [25] was used in 79 Swedish patients (mean age 48 years), giving an 80% complete remission rate, of whom 17% have relapsed, leading to a 58% disease-free survival after a median follow up of 8 months. The toxicity was severe, with 59% developing moderate or severe mucositis. Initially, no prophylactic antibiotic treatment was given, and during this period there were 7 lethal pulmonary infections. Thus, prophylaxis with antibiotics seems important.

It was concluded that randomised trials are needed to evaluate the efficacy of MACOP-B and other third-generation combination chemotherapies compared to conventional CHOP and CHOP-like regimens.

Bone Marrow Transplantation in High-Grade Malignant Non-Hodgkin's Lymphoma

High-dose chemotherapy with or without TBI followed by ABMT has proven to salvage 10-

20% of end-stage patients with refractory or relapsed high-grade malignant lymphoma, giving emphasis to such an approach [26]. Experimental animal data [27] and clinical studies [28] suggest a dose-dependent response of lymphoma cells to chemotherapy, making this disease group suitable for high-dose treatment with marrow rescue. However, it is more difficult to evaluate the utility of ABMT in lymphoma than in acute myeloid leukaemia. Firstly, as yet no randomised trials with ABMT are available. Secondly, the heterogeneity of lymphomas regarding histology and clinical staging is adding to the difficulties in evaluating the data. Thirdly, the prognostic features emerging from studies with CHOP or CHOP-like therapies are not necessarily applicable to patients receiving third-generation front-line therapy.

Indications

The most important point of discussion is which patients should be transplanted. The optimal benefit of ABMT would be to treat patients with early disease who do well with ABMT but would have relapsed if given conventional therapy. However, this patient group is not easily identified. Patients with complete remission after 3 courses of CHOP have a good prognosis without ABMT, whereas those who do not respond at all to first-line therapy will also do badly after an ABMT. The main groups would probably be poor prognosis patients in first complete remission, such as those with lymphoblastic lymphomas with previous bone marrow or central nervous system involvement; furthermore patients with partial remission after intensive first-line therapy, and also relapsed patients with tumours that are still responsive to therapy. Some centres advocate ABMT in first remission for all patients with lymphoblastic lymphomas due to an experience of poor prognosis for these patients despite aggressive initial treatment, such as that reported by Coleman et al. [29].

Results

The greatest knowledge on ABMT in lymphoma emerges from the retrospective registry data of the European Cooperative Group for Bone Marrow Transplantation (EBMT) [30]. It comprises 393 adults and 118 children with intermediate or high-grade lymphoma, of which half had a relapse or had never entered a complete remission whereas one-fourth were treated in first complete remission. The projected 5-year disease-free survival of patients in complete remission after ABMT was 56%, significantly better for adults than for children and also significantly related to disease status at ABMT. The histology and initial stage of the lymphomas seemed to be of less importance for the outcome.
The ABMT-procedure-related overall mortality was 17%, with a significant association to the disease status at transplant; 9% toxic deaths among those who were transplanted in first complete remission compared to 20% in those treated in relapse.

Methods

Total body irradiation. The use of TBI in the preparative regimen is questionable. It gives a higher procedure-related mortality and chemotherapy programmes without TBI permit the use of radiotherapy to sites of bulky disease [31].
Purging of bone marrow in vitro. There is much debate on the usefulness of purging the autologous bone marrow *in vitro* before reinfusion. The purging is mostly performed with monoclonal antibodies with different B-cell specificities and complement. In the EBMT registry data bone marrow involvement did not influence outcome in lymphoblastic lymphoma patients. When testing the effects of purging by univariate analysis, there was a borderline significance in favour of purging. However, this difference was not reproduced in multivariate analyses when other prognostic factors were considered. The Seattle group have compared the results in lymphoma transplants according to the source of the marrow (syngeneic, allogeneic, or autologous) and found no influence on disease-free survival or probability of relapse [32]. Clinical data arguing against purging are the finding that most relapses occur at previous bulky disease [31]; 70% of the relapses occur at old sites of lymphoma involvement with or without new sites as well, whereas only 10% of these

relapses occur in new sites only. However, 20% of the relapses occur in blood and bone marrow for the first time. It seems clear that the major problem with the lymphoma transplants is to eradicate the malignant cells from the patients, whereas the clearing of lymphoma cells from the bone marrow with specific methods is, at present, a less pressing matter. It has been suggested that the transplant procedure (aspirating, freezing and thawing) of itself reduces the number of clonogenic lymphoma cells in the reinfused marrow. It is also possible that the "take" within the spongeous bone may favour the normal stem cells compared with the clonogenic tumour cells. Furthermore, the so-called specific purging methods can only reduce the number of cells carrying the phenotype corresponding to that of the majority of the tumour cells, but this phenotype is not likely to be equivalent to the phenotype of the clonogenic tumour cells, which are those that are crucial to eradicate.

Autologous versus allogeneic bone marrow transplantation. The EBMT data were also used for a comparison between autologous versus allogeneic bone marrow transplantation. There were no significant differences in overall survival, remission rate or relapse rate. However, the allogeneic transplant patients were younger. A graft-versus-lymphoma activity could not be confirmed, nor excluded. Graft-versus-host disease was the major cause of the higher procedure-related death rate in allogeneic compared to autologous bone marrow transplants: 31% and 17%, respectively. The upper age limit is higher for autologous than for allogeneic transplants (about 60 years and 43 to 50 years, respectively). These findings favour the autologous procedure in cases without residual bone marrow disease. However, the comparisons made were not strict in many respects, and it was pointed out that the procedure-related deaths of allogeneic transplants can be reduced by using more effective prophylaxis against graft-versus-host disease, such as T-cell depletion of the marrow or the combination of cyclosporin A and methotrexate. Further trials are needed to evaluate the role of allogeneic as well as autologous bone marrow transplants in lymphoma.

REFERENCES

1 Horning SJ, Rosenberg SA: The natural history of initially untreated low-grade non-Hodgkin's lymphomas. N Engl J Med 1984 (311):1471-1475

2 Yunis JJ, Frizzera G, Oken MM, McKenna J, Theologides A, Arnesen M: Multiple recurrent genomic defects in follicular lymphoma. A possible model for cancer. N Engl J Med 1987 (316):79-84

3 Gahrton G, Lindsten J, Zech L: Involvement of chromosomes 8, 9, 19 and 22 in Ph1 positive and Ph1 negative chronic myelocytic leukemia in the chronic and blastic stage. Acta Med Scand 1974 (196):355-360

4 Rowley JD: Ph1 positive leukaemia including chronic myelogeneous leukaemia. Clin Haematol 1980 (9):55-86

5 Juliusson G, Friberg K, Gahrton G: Consistency of chromosomal aberrations in chronic lymphocytic leukemia. A longitudinal study of 41 patients. Cancer 1988 (62):500-506

6 Bakhshi A, Jensen JP, Goldman P et al: Cloning the chromosomal breakpoint of t(14;18) human lymphomas: clustering around J_H on chromosome 14 and near a transcriptional unit on 18. Cell 1985 (41):899-906

7 Stansfeld AG, Diebold J, Kapanci Y, Kelényi G, Lennert K, Mioduszewska O, Noel H, Rilke F, Sundström C, Van Unnik JAM, Wright DH: Updated Kiel classification for lymphomas. Lancet 1988 (i):292-293

8 Somers R, Burgers JMV, Qasim M, van Glabbeke M, Duez N, Hayat M: EORTC trial non-Hodgkin's lymphomas. Eur J Cancer Clin Oncol 1987 (23):283-293

9 Filly RA, Blank N, Castellino RA: Radiographic distribution of intrathoracic disease in previously untreated patients with Hodgkin's disease and non-Hodgkin's lymphoma. Radiology 1976 (120):277

10 Reznek RH, Richards MA: The radiology of lymphoma. In: Bailliere's Clinical Hematology 1987 (1):77-108

11 Bartl R, Frisch B, Burkhardt R (eds) Bone Marrow Biopsies Revisited. S. Karger, Basle 1985

12 Lindemalm C, Mellstedt H, Nilsson B, Biberfeld P, Björkholm M, Christensson B, Holm G, Johansson B: Blood clonal B cell excess (CBE) at diagnosis in patients with non-Hodgkin's lymphoma (NHL). Relation to clinical stage, histopathology and response to treatment. Eur J Cancer 1987 (23):749-753

13 Goffinet DR, Warnke R, Dunnick NR et al: Clinical and surgical (laparotomy) evaluation of patients with non-Hodgkin's lymphomas. Cancer Treat Rep 1977 (61):881-922

14 Lindgren PG, Hagberg H, Eriksson B, Glimelius B, Magnusson A, Sundström C: Excision biopsy of the spleen by ultrasonic guidance. Br J Radiol 1985 (58):653-657

15 Lewin KJ, Rachod M, Dorfman RF: Lymphomas of the gastrointestinal tract - a study of 117 cases presenting with gastrointestinal disease. Cancer 1978 (42):693-707

16 Caletti GC, Lorenza Z, Bolondi L, Guizzardi G, Brocchi E, Barbara L: Impact of endoscopic ultrasonography on diagnosis and treatment of primary gastric lymphoma. Surgery 1988 (103):315-320
17 Hoerni-Simon G, Suchaud JP, Eghbali H, Coindre JM, Hoerni B: Secondary involvement of the central nervous sytem in malignant non-Hodgkin's lymphoma. A study of 30 cases in a series of 498 patients. Oncology 1987 (44):98-101
18 Parvinen LM, Jereb B, Nisce L: Primary non-Hodgkin's lymphoma ('reticulum cell sarcoma') of bone in adults. Acta Radiol Oncol 1983 (22):449-454
19 French Cooperative Group on CLL (chairman J-L Binet): A randomized comparison of no treatment versus daily chlorambucil in 612 patients with stage A CLL. (Abstract). 4th International Workshop on CLL, Paris 1988
20 Callagher CJ, Gregory WM, Jones AE et al: Follicular lymphoma: prognostic factors for response and survival. J Clin Oncol 1986 (4):1470-1480
21 Leavitt RD, Ratanatharathorn V, Ozer H et al: Alpha-2b-interferon in the treatment of Hodgkin's disease and non-Hodgkin lymphoma. Semin Oncol 1987 (14 suppl 2):18-23
22 Young RC, Longo DL, Glatsein E, Matis LA, Ostchega Y, Nanfro J, DeVita VR Jr: Watchful waiting versus aggressive combined modality therapy in the treatment of stage III-IV indolent non-Hodgkin's lymphoma. Proc Ann Meeting Am Soc Clin Oncol 1987 (6):A790
23 Knospe WH, Loeb V, Hugley CM: Biweekly chlorambucil treatment of chronic lymphocytic leukemia. Cancer 1974 (33):555-562
24 McKelvey EM, Gottlieb JA, Wilson HE et al: Hydroxyldaunomycin (adriamycin) combination chemotherapy in malignant lymphoma. Cancer 1976 (38):1484-1493
25 Klimo P, Connors JM: MACOP-B chemotherapy for the treatment of diffuse large cell lymphomas. Ann Int Med 1985 (102):596-602
26 Singer CRJ, Goldstone AH: Clinical studies of ABMT in non-Hodgkin's lymphoma. Clin Haematol 1986 (15):105-150
27 Bruce WB, Meeker BG, Valeriote FA: Comparison of the sensitivity of normal haemopoietic and transplanted lymphoma colony-forming cells to chemotherapeutic agents administered in vivo. JNCI 1966 (36):233-245
28 Frei III E, Canellos GP: Dose: a critical factor in cancer chemotherapy. Am J Med 1980 (69):585-594
29 Coleman CN, Picozzi VJ, Cox RS et al: Treatment of lymphoblastic lymphoma in adults. J Clin Oncol 1986 (4):1628-1637
30 Goldstone AH, Gribben JG, Dones L: Fourth report of EBMT experience of autologous bone marrow transplantation in lymphoma. Bone Marrow Transpl 1987 (2 Suppl 1):200-203
31 Goldstone AH, Singer CRJ, Gribben JG, Jarrett M: Autologous bone marrow transplantation in lymphoma. Bone Marrow Transpl 1988 (in press)
32 Appelbaum FR, Sullivan KM, Buckner CD, Clift RA, Deeg HJ, Fefer A, Hill R, Mortimer J, Neiman PE, Sanders JE, Singer J, Stewart P, Storb R, Thomas ED: Treatment of malignant lymphoma in 100 patients with chemotherapy, total body irradiation, and marrow transplantation. J Clin Oncol 1987 (5):1340-1347

Present Indications and Results of Radiotherapy in Non-Hodgkin's Lymphomas

Mauro G. Trovò and Roberto Bortolus

Department of Radiotherapy, Centro di Riferimento Oncologico, Aviano, Italy

Non-Hodgkin's Lymphomas (NHL) are a very complex group of diseases and there are many reasons which prevent the physician from confidently being able to base management decisions on published data from studies on NHL. The choice of treatment requires a balancing of radiation therapy (RT) with systemic chemotherapy (CT). In some cases, RT alone may be sufficient, whereas in the presence of advanced disease or of unfavourable histologies a large number of patients have to be managed with CT, either alone or in combination with RT.

We must distinguish the major factors which influence management decisions, particularly because they affect the use of RT. The most significant factors are: extent of disease (stage), pathological subtype, bulk of disease, age of the patients and radiation dose [1-6]. Despite the confusion due to the different histopathological classifications [4,7], clinicians have tended to simplify the NHL subdivisions into two or three subgroups according to the apparent degree of malignancy or aggressiveness of the disease [5]. In this report, the indications and results of radiotherapy of NHL, according to stage and histology, are presented.

The Management of NHL Stage I and of Low-Grade Lymphoma Stage II

As reported in large series of patients, the incidence of stage I disease ranges from 12% to 20% and that of stage II disease from 18% to 25% (follicular histology < 10%, diffuse histology about 30%) [5,8-10]. At present, on the basis of the data reported in the literature, it is well defined that for stage I disease of nodular or diffuse histopathological subtype, radiation therapy alone is the standard management [1,11-13]. Histology is an important prognostic factor in NHL stage I; in fact, an analysis of the most recent data published shows that for follicular stage I disease, the long-term RFS following treatment by RT alone is approximately 50-60%, whereas for the diffuse pattern it is 45-50% [1].

The 1970-1975 LR1 EORTC trial compared mantle field RT (uninvolved mediastinum, not irradiated) with or without irradiation of para-aortic lymph nodes in NHL stage I (follicular and diffuse histology). No difference in relapse-free and total survival was observed between the two arms [1].

The 1975-1980 LR2 EORTC trial compared RT (extended field) either alone or followed by 12 cycles of adjuvant CT with cyclophosphamide, vincristine, prednisone (CVP). Among the 124 stage I patients the relapse-free interval was superior in the group receiving adjuvant CT (75% vs 55% at 5 years, $p < 0.002$) [14].

The 1975-1980 LR2 EORTC trial compared, in clinical or pathological stage II patients, RT to the involved side of the diaphragm alone with RT to both sides (total nodal irradiation with abdominal bath). All patients were given 12 cycles of CVP thereafter. No significant difference between extended-field or total nodal irradiation was observed either in 4-year RFS (39% vs 54%) or in total survival (36% vs 55%). Primary radiotherapy followed by adjuvant CT was disappointing for patients with diffuse histology in stage II (4-year survival

10%), whereas it gave good survival (4-year survival 75%) for patients with follicular or partly follicular cell pattern (stage II) [14]. From this trial it was concluded that extended field RT is an adequate treatment in stage I and II patients of a favourable histological type, following pathological or clinical staging. Moreover, RT alone may also be adequate for pathological stage I patients with unfavourable histologies.

These data are comparable to those obtained by other important institutions: Stanford University and Princess Margaret Hospital, Toronto. Paryani et al. [15] reported the Stanford experience on 124 stage I-II low-grade lymphoma patients treated with involved, extended or total lymphoid fields. Ten-year freedom from relapse was 54% and 10-year survival 68%. These results are very similar to those reported by Gospodarowicz et al. [16] on 190 patients from the Princess Margaret Hospital. Ten-year freedom from relapse and 10-year survival were 53% and 58%, respectively. The analysis of the Stanford data indicates that patients younger than 40 years of age have a very good prognosis, whereas the Princess Margaret Hospital data indicate better survival for patients younger than 70 years of age who have two involved areas and no bulky disease > 5 cm diameter.

The Management of Aggressive NHL Stage II

Traditionally, before the introduction of effective combination CT, early-stage aggressive NHL was managed with RT. With correct staging and a good RT technique, RT alone, with extended or total lymphoid irradiation, can yield 5-year survival rates of 90% to 100% in stage I large-cell lymphoma [11,17,18], but the same good results cannot be obtained in stage II. The results with RT alone in clinical stage II aggressive NHL are disappointing, with 5-year survival rates varying from 34% to 56% [11,19-25].

The relatively high relapse rates in stage II lymphoma mostly in non-contiguous lymph node-bearing areas [6,26], have led to the use of CT either as an adjuvant following RT, or as primary treatment. The group from Milan [27] that compared regional RT alone with RT followed by combination CT (CVP), reported that in patients with nodular histology, adjuvant CT failed to affect both RFS and overall survival significantly, whereas it was able to improve the cure rate in pathological stage I-II NHL with diffuse histology.

The following study of the same group [28] showed in a randomised trial on stage I-II patients with diffuse histology the superiority of combination RT and the BACOP regimen versus RT and CVP.

In a randomised study of extended-field RT alone versus RT plus adjuvant CT with vincristine, streptonigrin, cyclophosphamide and prednisone in stage I-II NHL, Nissen [29] concluded by recommending the use of adjuvant CT with RT in all stage I-II patients with unfavourable histology. In fact, CT improved both relapse-free and overall survival. The same conclusions were reached by Landberg [30] in a randomised multicentre study using adjuvant CVP. Encouraging results were reported by Cosset et al. [31] with an alternating CT and RT combination for unfavourable histologies. Long-term results are needed to confirm these preliminary data.

The Eastern Cooperative Oncology Group (ECOG) [32] confirmed that combination CT with the COPA regimen, followed by moderate dose (25-30 Gy in 2-3 weeks) involved-field RT in complete responders with clinical stage II or II E aggressive histological NHL can produce a good survival (86%) at 4 years. The ECOG is currently comparing in selected patients with stage I and II aggressive disease CT alone with CT followed by consolidation RT for complete responders.

In contrast with the above-mentioned reports, the BNLI [24] found no benefit combining chlorambucil or COP with regional RT and also the Stanford experience of adjuvant CAT or COP following total nodal irradiation in pathological stage I-II diffuse NHL found no benefit with the combined approach [33].

In summary, the available data would indicate that radiation therapy alone is probably not the optimal treatment for diffuse histology stage II patients. Combination CT seems to be very effective and to induce remission; however, relapses still occur in initially involved sites. The optimal extent of irradiation and its combination with CT deserves further investigation.

The Management of NHL Stage III and IV

Histological grade, follicular or diffuse architectural pattern is more important than the distinction between stage III and IV for patients with advanced NHL. Despite a large number of clinical trials in the last two decades, the treatment of patients with low-grade advanced disease remains controversial.

In the EORTC trial (20751) [14], all stage III and IV patients were treated with 8 cycles of combination CT followed by local adjuvant RT in a total dose of 30 Gy (1.5 Gy per fraction) on the areas with initial disease greater than 5 cm or on the areas where the nodes were still present after 3 cycles of CT. The 5-year overall survival and RFS were 68% and 38%, respectively, for stage III-IV follicular lymphoma patients.

These results are very similar to those obtained at Stanford University with other treatments, such as a single alkylating agent or whole body irradiation plus boost, or CVP, or total lymphoid irradiation and CVP [34,35]. The Stanford results were unable to demonstrate a role for irradiation as an adjuvant to CT in patients with advanced-stage disease, either in low-grade or in large-cell lymphomas [11]. For some categories of patients (i.e., age > 40 years) with low-grade advanced NHL, the "wait and see" approach could be justified [36]. For stage III and stage IV diffuse lymphoma, aggressive CT regimens are considered the standard treatment. No data reported in the literature indicate a role for irradiation either as an adjuvant to chemotherapy or as the only treatment.

In the EORTC trial (20751) [14], 5-year relapse-free and overall survival rates of 19% and 30%, respectively, were reported for diffuse stage III-IV lymphoma. These results are similar to those reported in other studies using CHOP or CHOP-like regimens [37,38].

In the last decade, with the advent of more intensive regimens, higher complete remission and longer disease-free survival rates have been reported [39-48]. However, all the new CT regimens should be compared in randomised studies with CHOP [40].

The precise role of radiotherapy in central nervous system (CNS) prophylaxis has to be considered separately. As reported by Hoppe [11], the patients at greatest risk for CNS relapse are those with large-cell lymphoma showing bone marrow involvement, sinus involvement or testicular involvement and all patients with lymphoblastic lymphoma or undifferentiated lymphoma. Currently, a dose of 24 Gy in 2.5 weeks is delivered to the whole brain. The dose should be greater in the case of leptomeningeal involvement.

In conclusion, the important palliative role of irradiation should not be forgotten. Although aggressive treatment regimens are used in NHL, there are still many patients relapsing who can no longer be candidates for curative treatment programmes but who can benefit from RT. Moreover, NHL occurs frequently in elderly patients (> 70 years of age) and often the best treatment for these patients, who cannot be treated with standard aggressive CT, is radiation therapy.

REFERENCES

1 Tubiana M, Carde P, Burgers JMV, Cosset JM, Van Glabbeke M, Somers R: Prognostic factors in non-Hodgkin's lymphoma. Int J Radiat Oncol Biol Phys 1985 (12):503-514

2 Jones SE, Fuks Z, Kaplan HS, et al: Non-Hodgkin's lymphomas. Results of radiotherapy. Cancer 1973 (32):682

3 Carbone PP, Kaplan HS, Musshof K, et al: Report of the Committee on Hodgkin's disease staging classification. Cancer Res 1971 (31):1860

4 Rappaport H: Tumors of the hematopoietic system. In: Atlas of Tumor Pathology, section 3, Fasc. 8. Armed Forces Institute of Pathology, Washington 1966

5 The Non-Hodgkin's Lymphoma Pathologic Classification Project: National Cancer Institute sponsored study of classifications of non-Hodgkin's lymphomas: Summary and description of a working formulation for clinical usage. Cancer 1982 (49):2112

6 Fuks Z, Kaplan HS: Recurrence rates following radiation therapy of nodular and diffuse lymphomas. Radiology 1973 (108):675

7 Lukes RJ, Collins RD: New approaches to the classification of the lymphomata. Br J Cancer 1975 (3-Suppl 2):1

8 Castellani R, Bonadonna G, Spinelli R, Baietta E, Galante E, Rilke F: Sequential pathologic staging of untreated non-Hodgkin's lymphomas by laparoscopy and laparotomy combined with marrow biopsy. Cancer 1977 (40):2322-2328

9 Chabner BA, Johnson RE, Young RC, Canellos GP, Hubbard SP, Johnson SK, De Vita VT Jr: Sequential non surgical and surgical staging of non-Hodgkin's lymphomas. Ann Intern Med 1976 (85):149-154

10 Goffinet DR, Warnke R, Dunnick NR, Castellino R, Glatstein E, Nelsen PS, Dorfman RF, Rosenberg SA, Kaplan HS: Clinical and surgical (laparotomy) evaluation of patients with non-Hodgkin's lymphomas. Cancer Treat Rep 1977 (61):981-992

11 Hoppe RT: The role of radiation therapy in the management of the non-Hodgkin's lymphomas. Cancer 1985 (55):2176-2183

12 Sutcliffe SB, Gospodarowicz MK, Bush RS, Brown TC, Chua T, Bean HA, Clark RM, Dembo A, Fitzpatrick PJ, Peters MV: Role of radiation therapy in localized non-Hodgkin's lymphoma. Radiother Oncol 1985 (4):211-223

13 Glatstein E, Wasserman TH: Non-Hodgkin's Lymphomas. In: Perez C, Brady WL (eds) Principles and Practice of Radiation Oncology. JB Lippincott, Philadelphia 1987 pp 1073-1085

14 Somers R, Burgers JMV, Qasim M, Van Glabbeke M, Duez N, Hayat M: EORTC trial non-Hodgkin Lymphomas. Eur J Cancer Clin Oncol 1987 (23):283-293

15 Paryani SB, Hoppe RT, Cox RS, Colby TV, Rosenberg SA, Kaplan HS: Analysis of non-Hodgkin's lymphomas with nodular and favourable histologies, stage I and II. Cancer 1983 (52):2300-2307

16 Gospodarowicz MK, Bush RS, Brown TC, Chua T: Prognostic factors in nodular lymphomas: a multivariate analysis based on the Princess Margaret Hospital experience. Int J Radiat Oncol Biol Phys 1981 (10):489-497

17 Levitt SH, Bloomfield CD, Frizzera G, Lee CKK: Curative radiotherapy for localized diffuse histiocytic lymphoma. Cancer Treat Rep 1980 (64):175-177

18 Suit DL, Golomb HN: The treatment of histiocytic lymphoma. Semin Oncol 1980 (7):302-309

19 Bonadonna G, Lattuada A, Banfi A: Recent trends in the medical treatment of non-Hodgkin's lymphomas. Europ J Cancer 1976 (12): 661-673

20 Bush RS, Gospodarowicz M, Sturgeon J, Alison R: Radiation therapy of localized non-Hodgkin's lymphoma. Cancer Treat Rep 1977 (61):1129

21 Lamb DS, Vaughan Hudson G, Easterling MJ, MacLennan KA, Jelliffe AM: Localised grade 2 non-Hodgkin's lymphoma: results of treatment of radiotherapy (BNLI report n. 24). Clinical Radiol 1984 (35):253-260

22 Mill WB, Lee FA, Franssila KO: Radiation therapy of stage I and II extranodal non-Hodgkin's lymphoma of the head and neck. Cancer 1980 (45):653-661

23 Peckham MJ, Guay JP, Hamlin IME, Lukes RJ: Survival in localised nodal and extranodal non-Hodgkin's lymphomata. Br J Cancer 1975 (31):413-424

24 Phillips DL: Radiotherapy in the treatment of localised non-Hodgkin's lymphomas. (BNLI Report n. 16). Clin Radiol 1981 (32):543-546

25 Reddy S, Saxena VR, Pellettiere EV, Hendrickson FR: Early nodal and extranodal non-Hodgkin's lymphomas. Cancer 1977 (40):98-104

26 Fuks Z, Glatstein E, Kaplan HS: Patterns of presentation and relapse in the non-Hodgkin's lymphomata. Br J Cancer 1975 (31):286-297

27 Monfardini S, Banfi A, Bonadonna G, Rilke F, Milani F, Valagussa P, Lattuada A: Improved five year survival after combined radiotherapy-chemotherapy for stage I-II non-Hodgkin's lymphomas. Int J Radiat Oncol Biol Phys 1980 (6):125-134

28 Bajetta E, Valagussa P, Bonadonna G, Lattuada A, Buzzoni R, Rilke F, Banfi A: Combined modality treatment for stage I-II non-Hodgkin's lymphomas: CVP versus Bacop chemotherapy. Int J Radiat Oncol Biol Phys 1988 (15):3-12

29 Nissen NI, Ersboll J, Hansen HS, Walbom-Jorgensen S, Pedersen-Bjergaard J, Hansen MM, Rygard J: A randomized study of radiotherapy versus radiotherapy plus chemotherapy in stage I-II non-Hodgkin's lymphomas. Cancer 1983 (52):1-7

30 Landberg TG, Hakansson LG, Moller TR, Mattsson WKI, Landys KE, Johansson BG, Killander DCF, Molin BF, Westling PF, Lenner PH, Dahl OG: CVP-remission-maintenance in stage I or II non-Hodgkin's lymphomas. Preliminary results of a randomized study. Cancer 1979 (44):831-838

31 Cosset JM, Ozanne F, Henry-Amar M, Carde P, Amiel JL, Hayat M, Habrand JL, Tubiana M: An alternating chemotherapy and radiotherapy combination for non-Hodgkin's lymphomas of unfavourable histologies: feasibility and preliminary results. Radiother Oncol 1985 (3):133-138

32 O'Connell MJ, Harrington DP, Earle JD, Johnson GJ, Glick JH, Neiman RS, Silverstein MN: Chemotherapy followed by consolidation radiation therapy for the treatment of clinical stage II aggressive histologic type non-Hodgkin's lymphoma. Cancer 1988 (61):1754-1758
33 Glatstein E, Donaldson SS, Rosenberg SA, Kaplan HS: Combined modality treatment in malignant lymphomas. Cancer Treat Rep 1977 (61):1199-1207
34 Hoppe RT, Kushlan P, Rosenberg SA, Kaplan HS: The treatment of advanced stage favorable histology non-Hodgkin's lymphoma: a preliminary report of a randomized trial comparing single agent chemotherapy, combination chemotherapy, and whole body irradiation. Blood 1981 (58):592-598
35 Rosenberg SA: The low grade non-Hodgkin's lymphomas: challenges and opportunities. J Clin Oncol 1985 (3):299-310
36 Horning SJ, Rosenberg SA: The natural history of initially untreated low-grade non-Hodgkin lymphomas. New Engl J Med 1984 (311):1476-1481
37 McKelvey EM, Gottlieb JA, Wilson HE et al: Hydroxydaunomycin (adriamycin) combination chemotherapy in malignant lymphoma. Cancer 1976 (38):1484-1493
38 Fisher RI, Dahlberg S, Miller TP, Jones SE, Coltman CA: Long term survival of patients with nodular histiocytic (NH), diffuse poorly differentiated lymphocytic (DPDL), diffuse mixed (DM) and diffuse undifferentiated lymphoma treated with CHOP chemotherapy. Proceedings A.S.C.O. Vol. 8 March 1989, # 1003
39 Gordon LI, Harrington D, Glick JH, Colgan J, O'Connell M, Oken M, Resnick G, Anderson J, Gottlieb A for ECOG and CALGB: Randomized phase III comparison of CHOP vs m-BACOD in diffuse large cell (DH) and diffuse mixed (DM) lymphoma: equivalent complete response (CR) rates and time to treatment failure but greater toxicity with m-BACOD. Proceedings A.S.C.O. Vol. 8 March 1989, # 995
40 Wieck J, Dahlberg S, Miller T, Dana B, Fisher R: The treatment of non-Hodgkin's lymphoma with m-BACOD, ProMACE-CytaBOM, and MACOP-B: The Southwest Oncology Group (SWOG) experience. Proceeding A.S.C.O. Vol. 8 March 1989, # 990
41 Chisesi T, Santini G, Congiu A, Sertoli MR, Porcellini A, Rizzoli V, Coser P, Ardizzoni A, Contu A for the Italian NHL Cooperative Study Group (NHLCSG): Alternating promace/MOP chemotherapy in intermediate and high-grade diffuse non-Hodgkin's lymphomas (NHL). Proceedings A.S.C.O. Vol. 8 March 1989, # 1059
42 Jones SE, Salmon S, Fisher R: Adjuvant immunotherapy with BCG in non-Hodgkin's lymphoma: a Southwest Oncology Group controlled clinical trial. In: Jones SE, Salmon S (eds) Adjuvant Therapy of Cancer II. Grune and Stratton, New York 1979 pp 163-171
43 Canetta R et al: Sequential non-cross-resistant regimens (CVP and ABP) in advanced non-Hodgkin lymphomas. Proc Am Assoc Cancer Res 1980 (21):189
44 Laurence J et al: Combination chemotherapy of advanced diffuse histiocytic lymphoma with the six-drug COP-BLAM regimen. Annals of Internal Medicine 1982 (97):190-195
45 Skarin AT et al: Improved prognosis of diffuse histiocytic and undifferentiated lymphoma by use of high dose methotrexate alternating with standard agents (M-MACOD). J Clin Oncol 1983 (1):91-98
46 Fisher RI et al: Diffuse aggressive lymphomas: increased survival after alternating flexible sequences of ProMACE and MOP chemotherapy. Ann Int Med 1983 (98):304-309
47 Cabanillas F et al: Sequential chemotherapy and late intensification for malignant lymphomas of aggressive histologic type. Am J Med 1983 (74):382-388
48 Connors JM, Klimo P: Cancer Control Agency of British Columbia Vancouver, BC Canada V5Z 3J3 1984 MACOP-B treatment of advanced diffuse large cell lymphoma 1984
49 Tirelli U, Zagonel V, Serraino D, Thomas J, Hoerni B, Tanguri A, Ruhl , Bey P, Tubiana M, Breed WPM, Roozendaal KJ, Hagenbeek A, Hupperets PS, Somers R: Non-Hodgkin's lymphomas in 137 patients aged 70 years or older: a retrospective European Organization for Research and Treatment of Cancer Lymphoma Group Study. J Clin Oncol 1988 (6):1708-1713

Treatment of Childhood Non-Hodgkin's Lymphomas: Trends in Europe

Catherine Patte

Department of Paediatrics, Institut Gustave-Roussy, Villejuif, France

In the past decade, there have been major advances in the treatment of children with non-Hodgkin's lymphoma (NHL). On the one hand, biological and immunological characterisation has contributed significantly to our understanding of these disorders. On the other, the observation that lymphomas are a heterogeneous group of diseases with differing clinical presentations and histological subgroups and, above all, optimal response to different treatment regimens, has led to better schemes of treatment based on intensive polychemotherapy.

Generalities on Childhood NHL

Before dealing with treatment, some generalities have to be recalled: 1) Childhood NHLs are diffuse high-grade malignancies. In the Kiel classification [1], which is most commonly used in Europe, the majority are classified as lymphoblastic, a group which is subdivided into lymphoblastic or Burkitt's type (classified as undifferentiated or small non-cleaved in the Rappaport, or in the Working Formulation [2]), lymphoblastic with convoluted nuclei, and lymphoblastic non-Burkitt's, non-convoluted (lymphoblastic "other").
2) Immunophenotyping studies have shown that about 50% of the childhood NHLs are B-cell tumours expressing monoclonal immunoglobulin molecules on their surface, about 40% are derived from cells of T-lineage, and about 5% are non-T non-B derived neoplasms.
3) Histology has been found to correlate strongly with immunophenotype, which correlates strongly with clinical presentation [3-6]: the abdominal NHLs originating in the GI tract are B-cell lymphomas, usually classified as Burkitt's. The mediastinal NHLs originating in the anterior mediastinum have T-cell markers and are classified as lymphoblastic non-Burkitt's, typically with convoluted nuclei. In the other primaries, which are less frequent and very various, different histologies and immunophenotypes can be encountered, hence the necessity of immunophenotyping studies.
4) As the primaries are not very often nodal, the Ann Arbor staging classification is not suitable for childhood NHL. The usual staging classification used is Murphy's staging system [7] (Table 1). Localised tumours (stages I and II) are rare, although stage III represents about half or the childhood NHLs and stage IV (bone marrow and/or CNS initial involvement) represents about one-third.
5) The childhood NHLs are very aggressive tumours, proliferating locally and disseminating very rapidly, especially in bone marrow and CNS.
Therefore, the treatment should be considered as an emergency, for NHL can be life threatening, due to local invasion or metabolic disturbances. The initial management must be precise and adapted, because children are exposed to a large number of complications, especially metabolic. The tumour lysis syndrome must be treated preventively.

Table 1. Murphy's staging classification for childhood NHL [7]

Stage	Criteria for extent of disease
I	A single tumour (extranodal) or single anatomical area (nodal) with the exclusion of the mediastinum or abdomen
II	A single tumour (extranodal) with regional node involvement Two or more nodal areas on the same side of the diaphragm Two single (extranodal) tumours with or without regional node involvement on the same side of the diaphragm A primary gastrointestinal tract tumour, usually in the ileocaecal area, with or without involvement of associated mesenteric nodes only, grossly completely resected
III	Two single tumours (extranodal) on opposite sides of the diaphragm Two or more nodal areas above and below the diaphragm All the primary intrathoracic tumours (mediastinal, pleural, thymic) All extensive primary intra-abdominal disease, unresectable All paraspinal or epidural tumours, regardless of other tumour site(s)
IV	Any of the above with initial CNS and/or bone marrow involvement

General Principles of Therapy

By the end of the 1970s it became clear that two subgroups had a different evolution with the same treatment. In France, with the COPAD protocol, a pulse polychemotherapy regimen with prednisone, vincristine, cyclophosphamide and adriamycin, a higher event-free survival (EFS) of Burkitt's lymphomas was achieved than for lymphoblastic non-Burkitt's lymphomas: in the series of 204 patients treated at the Institut Gustave-Roussy from 1974 to 1980, EFS at 3 years was 52% (with a plateau at 14 months) and 19%, respectively [8-10].

In Germany, with the protocol BMF 76-81 for ALL, results were inverted: with this semicontinuous regimen EFS was 78% for non-localised non-B lymphoma [11].

The same conclusion was drawn from the CCSG randomised trial in the US, where two protocols were compared [12]: The COMP protocol, a 4-drug pulse regimen, and the LSA_2L_2 protocol, a 10-drug semicontinuous regimen, first described by Wollner [13] and developed originally at Memorial Sloan-Kettering Cancer Center as leukaemia therapy. This trial showed that, in patients with advanced disease, the effectiveness of both regimens was histology specific. The 2-year relapse-free survival rates for patients with non-localised lymphoblastic disease were: LSA_2L_2 76% and COMP 26%, compared to non-lymphoblastic disease: LSA_2L_2 28% and COMP 57% [14].

It was concluded that B-cell lymphomas need a short pulse intensive polychemotherapy regimen, whereas T-cell lymphomas need a longer semicontinuous polychemotherapy regimen as applied to high-risk leukaemia. The rare non-T non-B lymphomas are generally treated with the same protocol as T-cell lymphomas.

Localised lymphomas need less intensive treatment than non-localised lymphomas and CNS prophylaxis can be avoided in stage I and abdominal II [4,8,15]. As in the US [16,17], localised diseases are sometimes treated with a similar treatment, whatever the histology may be [18,19], but many groups in Europe think that localised disease should receive a treatment adapted to histology and immunology.

It is now widely admitted that, except in the case of very small tumours, for which excision is carried out at the same time as biopsy, surgery has no place in the treatment of childhood NHL. There is no indication for removal of an extended tumour to be attempted; the surgical excision leads to useless mutilation which delays chemotherapy and may even complicate it.

Although childhood NHL is very radiosensitive and locally radiocurable, irradiation is no longer performed because it does not prevent tumour extension outside of the radiation field and it adds significantly to treatment morbidity, without any demonstrable benefit. Therefore, indications for local irradiation are generally restricted to a few residual masses after induction.

As remission duration has improved, the central nervous system as a site of relapse has become increasingly important and the improvement of CNS prophylaxis a matter of great concern. The CNS prophylaxis which proved effective in lymphoblastic leukaemias was first used: radiotherapy on the skull with intrathecal chemotherapy, or intrathecal drugs alone. Yet, a certain percentage of failures and the neuroendocrine long-term sequelae of cranial irradiation led to a search for less toxic and more efficient therapy: HD MTX has become a drug of choice for CNS prophylaxis and has been included in several protocols.

Treatment of B-Type Lymphomas

Whenever possible, B-type NHL is defined by tumour cell immunophenotyping. It includes Burkitt's-type lymphoblastic, lymphoblastic B non-Burkitt's, centroblastic and most immunoblastic lymphomas. Primarily, intra-abdominal lymphomas are considered as B-type despite inconclusive histology and/or immunology, since a primary site in the abdomen is highly specific of B-type NHL.

In 1981, the French group SFOP (Société Française d'Oncologie Pédiatrique) and the German BFM group initiated, simultaneously, intensive pulse polychemotherapy regimens for B-cell lymphomas in multicentre studies.

The SFOP LMB Protocols

A pilot study, the LMB 01.81 protocol, on 32 patients, was highly efficient, but too toxic, and a few modifications led to the LMB 02.81 protocol [20]. This protocol was used in a multicentre study on patients with advanced stages (i.e., nasopharyngeal stages II, III and IV) from November 1981 to March 1984. It was a 9-drug pulse intensive polychemotherapy regimen over a period of one year, based on the use of high-dose cyclophosphamide (1.5 g/m^2 and 3 g/m^2 in the first and second induction courses), HD MTX (3g/m^2 in 3-hour infusion) and Ara-C in continuous infusion during 2 consolidation phases. CNS prophylaxis was performed with chemotherapy alone and based particularly on HD MTX, followed by intrathecal injections of MTX. No irradiation was performed. This study on 114 children with stages III and IV has been reported [20]. The conclusions were: 1) the overall and event-free survival were much improved: 73% (SE 5) for 72 stage III and 76% (SE 8) for the 21 stage IV patients without CNS involvement; 2) CNS prophylaxis was very efficient, with an isolated CNS relapse rate of 1%; 3) as with previous, less intensive treatments, relapse still occurred only during the first year; 4) the toxic death rate was too high, namely, 10%; 5) two bad prognostic factors were: the absence of complete remission (CR) after the third induction course, requiring an intensification of treatment by high-dose polychemotherapy and bone marrow transplantation to obtain a cure, and initial CNS involvement with an EFS of only 19% (SE 8) in 21 patients. Nine patients with extensive nasopharyngeal stage II tumours were also treated according to that protocol with a 100% EFS.

The following study, with the LMB84 protocol, was a randomised trial to study the possibility of reducing the length of treatment and, in consequence, the toxicity, without jeopardising the survival rates. The same patients were included, with the exception of those with CNS involvement [21]. All patients received the same 3 induction courses, which were similar to those of the LMB 02.81 protocol, with the omission of asparaginase. If CR was achieved, the patient was randomised between an 8-drug long arm, with 5 more courses, similar to the LMB 02.81, but a total treatment of 7 months, and a 6-drug short arm with 2 more courses to a total treatment of 4 months. In the case of partial remission, chemotherapy was intensified. Two hundred and sixteen patients from 27 French, one Belgian and one Dutch centres were registered between April 1984 and September 1987 (last randomisation: December 1987): 15 nasopharyngeal and facial, stage II, 167 stage III and 34 stage IV, 20 of which having more than 25% blast cells in bone marrow.

The primary site of involvement was abdomen in 172, head and neck in 30, thorax in 2 and other sites in 12. One hundred and sixty-seven patients are alive in first CR with a minimum follow up of 12 months. Eight patients died from initial tumour failure, 14 died from toxicity or deaths unrelated to tumour or treatment, 27 relapsed. With a median follow up of 38 months, EFS is 78% (SE 3) for all patients, 73% (SE 11) for the stage II patients, 80% (SE 3) for the stage III patients and 68% (SE 8) for the stage IV and ALL patients. One hundred and sixty-six patients were randomised: 82 in the short arm and 84 in the long arm. EFS is 89% and 87%, respectively. The statistical analysis of equivalence concludes in equivalence of both arms in terms of EFS rate. Moreover, morbidity was decreased in the short arm.

Since the end of randomisation all patients are treated according to the short arm. The aim of the next study will be to find prognostic factors suggested by the study; a further step would be to try to diminish the intensity of treatment for a group of patients and to select early the small group of patients who would need an intensified treatment.

For NHL with initial CNS involvement and for B-ALL without head and neck and abdominal tumours, the LMB86 protocol was initiated in October 1985 [22]. The first 2 courses are the same as in the other LMB protocols, but with a higher dose of methotrexate (8g/m^2 in 4-hour infusion) and with 9 triple intrathecal injections. Two consolidation courses are as follows: Ara-C 50 mg/m^2 in 12-hour continuous infusion day 1,2,3,4,5, followed by a boost of 3 g/m^2 in 3 hours day 2,3,4,5 and VP16 200 mg/m^2 day 2,3,4,5. They are followed by 4 less intensive maintenance courses, and 24 Gy cranial irradiation is performed during the first course. An optional arm with HD polychemotherapy + TBI, or craniospinal irradiation followed by bone marrow transplantation (BMT) after the first or second consolidation course is chosen by some centres. In November 1988, the EFS of 35 patients was 80% with a plateau at 9 months, 75% for 21 patients with NHL or ALL and initial CNS involvement and 85% for 14 patients with ALL and no CNS involvement. No difference has been observed so far between the grafted and the non-grafted patients, so the series will be continued without BMT.

Localised B-type lymphoma: although not registered in the LMB84 trial, all the other non-abdominal stage II patients were treated according to the short arm of the LMB84 protocol.

The patients with stage I or abdominal stage II NHL received the COPAD protocol without CNS prophylaxis for a period of 6 months. They were not registered nationally. The patients treated at the Institut Gustave-Roussy are all alive.

The BFM Protocols

Since 1981, B-type lymphomas and B-ALL have been treated by specific protocols [11]; there have been 3 successive studies: 81-83, 83-86 and 87, based on the same general scheme. After a 5-day cytoreductive phase with prednisone and cyclophosphamide, the patients received 2 alternative chemotherapy blocks. In the 1981-83 study, both blocks were given 5-day fractionated cyclophosphamide, intermediate-dose methotrexate (500 mg/m^2 in 24-hour infusion followed by leukovorin rescue 48 hours after the start of MTX infusion) and intrathecal methotrexate; VM26 and Ara-C alternated with adriamycin. Prednisone was continued for one month. The patients with localised tumour (i.e., stages I and resected stages II) received 4 blocks; those with advanced stage (i.e., non-resected stages II, III, IV and ALL) received 8 blocks, theoretically within 20 weeks, and prophylactic CNS irradiation. In the 1983-86 study, the regimen was slightly modified: prednisone was replaced by dexamethasone, intensified local chemotherapy in CNS disease at diagnosis, therapy reduced to 3 blocks in localised disease and 6 blocks in advanced disease [23]. In the 1987 study, which is still going on, ifosfamide replaces cyclophosphamide in one block, adriamycin, VM26 and Ara-C are fractionated, CNS irradiation is suppressed and, for stage IV and B-ALL, MTX is given at the dosage of 5 g/m^2 in 24-hour infusion.

These protocols improved prognosis substantially. The results of the combined trials 81-86 reported at the Third International Conference on Malignant Lymphoma in

Lugano, Switzerland, were: EFS 97% for 30 stage I patients, 90% for 23 resectable stage II patients, 90% for 26 non-resectable stage II patients, 73% for 75 stage III patients, 57% for 15 stage IV patients and 49% for 46 B-ALL (defined as more than 25% blast cells in bone marrow).

In Italy

Contrary to the trend with regard to ALL and Hodgkin's disease, there is no national study for childhood NHL. Some centres have adopted the BFM protocol, others the Murphy Total Therapy B presented at the 1983 ASCO meeting and published in 1986 [24]. This latter alternated 4 courses of fractionated cyclophosphamide, adriamycin, vincristine and triple intrathecal injections with 4 courses of HD MTX (1 g/m^2 in 24-hour infusion) followed by Ara-C 400 mg/m^2 during the next 48 hours. Ara-C was doubled in successive courses up to 3.2 g/m^2.
One centre, the *Istituto Nazionale Tumori* of Milan, developed its own protocol. Treatment in the first 5 weeks consisted of sequential weekly administration of vincristine + cyclophosphamide, HD MTX (100 mg/kg), adriamycin, HD MTX (150 mg/kg), vincristine. Following one week's rest, Ara-C 6 g/m^2 and CDDP 80 mg/m^2 were given in 96-hour continuous infusion. After recovery, 3 additional courses of chemotherapy (VCR+CPM, HD MTX 200 mg/m^2, VCR+ADM) completed the treatment programme. Eight i.t. injections of MTX and Ara-C were administered during the treatment. In 1987, at the Lugano conference, the results in 22 patients (1 stage I, 13 stage III and 8 stage IV) were: 2 early deaths from sepsis, 19 CR, 5 relapses, 14 alive in first CR, EFS 66% [25].

Treatment of Non-B-Type Lymphoma

This group includes lymphomas having T-cell markers, or non-T non-B-cell markers in immunophenotyping studies. They are generally classified as lymphoblastic non-Burkitt's lymphoma. Most of them have mediastinal involvement. These patients are generally treated with the same protocols as high-risk forms of acute lymphoblastic leukaemia.

The BFM Protocols and Derived Protocols

Since 1976, in the BFM studies, non B-type lymphomas received the same protocol as acute lymphoblastic leukaemias [11]. Localised diseases received a less intensive treatment, without cranial irradiation and without reinduction (protocol III or II). But all lymphomas received the same induction with protocol I, which underwent very few modifications during the studies, and a maintenance with daily 6-MP and weekly methotrexate. In the ongoing 1987 study, induction is followed by protocol M, a 57-day phase with 4 HD MTX (5 g/m^2 in 24-hour infusion) and i.t. MTX and daily purinethol; the total duration of treatment is 18 months. Since 1976, the results are about the same, since regimens were similar in the successive studies. The published stage III and IV EFS was 78% for 42 patients treated in the 75-81 study and 79% for 33 patients treated in the 81-83 study.
Now, several European groups and centres are following the BFM protocol, or slightly modified protocols [26,27]: the French-Belgian EORTC group, which since 1983 has been using a BFM-like protocol, the EORTC 58832 protocol for childhood ALL, now includes non-B-cell in the protocol; some Italian centres also treat NHL with the BFM protocol.

The LSA_2L_2 Protocol and Derived Protocols

The LSA_2L_2 protocol [13] is a 10-drug, intensive therapeutic regimen, with administration of drugs 5 days a week during consolidation, and 5 days every 2 weeks during maintenance to a total of 2 years, in general. Nevertheless, it can be administered in outpatient clinics. CNS prophylaxis is based on i.t. MTX.
This protocol has been tested by several groups and centres in Europe, which came to the following conclusions: 1) As shown by the CCSG randomised trial [12], the LSA_2L_2 protocol is efficient in mediastinal or lym-

phoblastic non-Burkitt's lymphomas, but not in abdominal lymphomas [28-32]; 2) CNS prophylaxis should be improved [33-37].
Vecchi [31] in Italy reported a series of patients for whom CNS prophylaxis was much improved by the addition of cranial irradiation. This modified protocol is still in progress. At the Institut Gustave-Roussy [34,35], the original protocol was modified by the addition of 10 HD MTX at the dosage of 3 g/m^2 in 3-hour infusion: 2 during induction, 3 during consolidation and 5 during maintenance. The EFS of 71 patients was 75% with a median follow up of 36 months and no relapse has occurred in the 65 patients with no initial CNS involvement. In France, this protocol was followed by many centres and a new study with a second generation LSA_2L_2 protocol will begin with a national registration.

Other Protocols

In France, several centres have included the non-B NHLs in the Fralle study conducted by the St. Louis Hospital for ALL [38].

Conclusion

Although they are aggressive diffuse malignancies, survival in childhood NHLs has greatly improved in the past 10 years. This is due to a better knowledge of the disease and to histology-adapted intensive polychemotherapy regimens. It is also due to a clinical research based on successive multicentre studies.
With the described regimens, EFS is now between 80% and 100% for localised disease and between 70% and 80% for extensive disease. It will not be easy to improve these results. The challenge for the coming years will be to try and diminish treatment, and therefore morbidity and sequelae, without jeopardising survival rates, for most patients, and to select the small group of bad-prognosis patients who need more intensive treatment.

REFERENCES

1 Lennert K, Mohri N: Histopathology and diagnosis of non-Hodgkin's lymphomas. In: Lennert K et al (eds) Malignant Lymphomas Other than Hodgkin's Disease. Springer Verlag, New York, 1978

2 National Cancer Institute-sponsored study of classification of non-Hodgkin's lymphomas: Summary and description of a working formulation for clinical usage. Cancer 1982 (49):2112-2135

3 Bernard A, Boumsell L, Bayle C et al: Subsets of malignant lymphomas in children related to the cell phenotype. Blood 1979 (54):1058-1068

4 Lemerle J, Bernard A, Patte C et al: Malignant B-cell lymphomas of childhood. In: Barrett A, Bloom HJG, Lemerle J et al (eds) Cancer in Children. Clinical Management (2nd edition). UICC Handbook, Springer Verlag, Heidelberg 1986 pp 37-51

5 Amylon MD, Link MP and Murphy SB: Malignant T-cell and other non-Hodgkin's lymphoma. In: Barrett A, Bloom HJG, Lemerle J et al (eds) Cancer in Children. Clinical Management (2nd edition). UICC Handbook, Springer Verlag, Heidelberg 1986 pp 152-163

6 Patte C, Bernard A, Bayle C: Lymphomes malins non Hodgkiniens. Med Infant 1988 (8):817-834

7 Murphy SB, Hustu HO: A randomized trial of combined modality therapy of childhood non-Hodgkin's lymphoma. Cancer 1980 (45):630-637

8 Patte C, Rodary C, Sarrazin D et al: Résultat du traitement de 178 lymphomes malins non Hodgkiniens de l'enfant de 1973 à 1978. Arch Fr Pediatr 1981 (38):321-327

9 Lemerle J: The treatment of B-cell non-Hodgkin's malignant lymphomas of childhood in Europe. Recent and on-going studies. In: Lenoir JM, O'Connor G, Olweny CLM (eds) Burkitt's Lymphoma, a Human Cancer Model. IARC Scient Publ No 60, Lyon 1985 pp 383-398

10 Philip T, Lenoir GM, Bryon PA et al: Burkitt type malignant lymphoma in France: individualisation among caucasian childhood non-Hodgkin's lymphoma. Br J Cancer 1982 (45):670-678

11 Muller-Weirich ST, Henze G, Odenwald E et al: BFM trials for childhood non-Hodgkin's lymphoma. In: Cavalli F, Bonadonna G, Rozencweig G (eds): Malignant Lymphomas and Hodgkin's Disease: Experimental and Therapeutic Advances. Martinus Nijhoff, Boston 1985 pp 633-642

12 Anderson JR, Wilson JR, Jenkin DT: Childhood non-Hodgkin's lymphoma: results of a randomized therapeutic trial comparing a 4-drug regimen (COMP) to a 10-drug regimen (LSA2L2). N Engl J Med 1983 (308):559-565

13 Wollner N, Exelby PR, Lieberman PH: Non-Hodgkin's lymphomas in children. A progress report on the original patients treated with the LSA2L2 protocol. Cancer 1979 (44):1990-1999

14 Jenkin RDT, Anderson JR, Chilcote RR, Coccia P, Exelby P, Kersey J, Kjeldsberg CR, Kushner J, Meadows AT, Siegel S, Wilson JF, Hammond D: The treatment of diffuse undifferentiated non-Hodgkin's lymphoma in children: the children's cancer study group experience. In: Lenoir JM, O'Connor G, Olweny CLM (eds) Burkitt's Lymphoma, a Human Cancer Model. IARC Scient Publ No 60, Lyon 1985 pp 399-404

15 Murphy SB: Management of childhood non-Hodgkin's lymphoma. Cancer Treat Rep 1977 (61):1161-1173

16 Jenkin RDT, Anderson JR, Chilcote RR, Coccia PF, Exelby PR, Kersey JH, Kushner JH, Meadows AT, Siegel SE, Wilson JF, Hammond GD: The treatment of localized non-Hodgkin's lymphoma in children: a report from the children's cancer study group. J Clin Oncol 1984 (2):88-97

17 Murphy SB, Hustu HO, Rivera G, Berard CW: End results of treating children with localized non-Hodgkin's lymphomas with a combined modality approach of lessened intensity. J Clin Oncol 1983 (1):326-330

18 Mott MG, Eden OB, Hann I for the UKCCSG: Curability of localised non-Hodgkin's lymphoma of childhood (NHL) without radiation. Med Ped Oncol 1988 (16):423 (abstract)

19 Gasparini M, Lombardi F, Fossati-Bellani F, Gianni C, Rottoli L: Localized non-Hodgkin's lymphoma (NHL) in children: results of a prospective treatment program including radiotherapy. Med Ped Oncol 1988 (16):421 (abstract)

20 Patte C, Philip T, Rodary C et al: Improved survival rate in children with stage III and IV B-cell non-Hodgkin's lymphoma and leukemia using multi-agent chemotherapy: results of a study of 114 children from the French Pediatric Oncology Society. J Clin Oncol 1986 (4):1219-1226

21 Patte C, Philip T, Rodary C, Zucker JM, Olive D, Béard C, Harousseau JL, Behrendt, Vannier JP, Pautard B, Demeocq F, for the SFOP: Updated results of the protocol LMB84 of the French Pediatriac Oncology Society (SFOP): randomized study to shorten duration of treatment of advanced stage B-cell non-Hodgkin's lymphoma (NHL) without CNS involvement. Med Ped Oncol 1988 (16):406 (abstract)

22 Patte C, Philip T, Zucker JM, Leverger G, Rubie H, Otten J, Benz-Lemoine E, on behalf of the SFOP: Results of the LMB86 protocol of the French Pediatric Oncology Society (SFOP) for B-cell non-Hodgkin's lymphoma (B-NHL) with CNS involvement (CNS+) and B-ALL. Proc ASCO J Clin Oncol 1989 (8) abstract No 1090

23 Müller-Weihrich ST, Ludwig R, Reiter A, Ritter J, Schrappe M, Riehm H: B-type non-Hodgkin's lymphomas and leukemia: the BFM study group experience. Proc of the Third International Conference on Malignant Lymphoma, Lugano 1987, abstract No 43, p 42

24 Murphy SB, Bowman WP, Abromowitch M, Mirro J, Ochs J, Rivera G, Pui CH, Fairclough D, Berard CW: Results of treatment of advanced-stage Burkitt's lymphoma and B-cell (Sig+) acute lymphoblastic leukemia with high-dose fractionated cyclophosphamide and coordinated high-dose methotrexate and cytarabine. J Clin Oncol 1986 (4):1732-1739

25 Gasparini M, Rottoli L, Gianni C, Morandi F, Ballerini E, Fossati-Bellani F: Intensive short-term chemotherapy for advanced childhood Burkitt-type

non-Hodgkin's lymphoma (B-NHL). Proc of the Third International Conference on Malignant Lymphoma, Lugano 1987, abstract No 47, p 44
26 Pacquement H, Asselin B, Quintana E, Dumont J, Mathiot C, Michon J, Zucker JM: Study of 24 children with non-B lymphoma treated in a single institution with a modified scheme of the German BFM. Med Ped Oncol 1988 (16):424 (abstract)
27 Guidicelli J, Bertrand Y, Paris A, Clerc M, Manel AM, Durin A: Treatment of malignant lymphomas with BFM-like regimen. Results about 12 cases. Med Ped Oncol 1988 (16):418 (abstract)
28 Pichler E, Jurgenssen O, Radaskiewicz T et al: Results of LSA2 L2 therapy in 26 children with non-Hodgkin's lymphoma. Cancer 1982 (50):2740-2746
29 Otten J, Benoit Y, Casteels-Vandaele M et al: Non-Hodgkin's lymphoma in children. A preliminary report of a study by the Belgian Cooperative Group for the treatment of solid tumours in children. Acta Pediatr Belg 1981 (34):157-164
30 Boguslawska-Jaworska J, Sonta-Jakimczyk D, Armata J, Rodziewicz B, Kazanowska B, Ochocka M, Rokicka-Milewska R, Radwanska U: The results of therapy in non-Hodgkin's lymphoma in children. A report on behalf of the Polish children's leukemia/lymphoma study group. Med Ped Oncol 1988 (16):419 (abstract)
31 Bezanilla Regato JL, Navajas A, Moya E, Lizarraga M: Modified LSA2L2 protocol in the treatment of twenty-six non-Hodgkin's lymphoma (NHL) children. Med Ped Oncol 1988 (16):442 (abstract)
32 Tzortzatou F, Mikraki V, Polychronopoulou S, Panayiotou J, Galanakis S, Vrachnou E, Tsomi K: Non-Hodgkin's lymphoma in childhood: a report of 49 cases. Med Ped Oncol 1988 (16):443 (abstract)
33 Vecchi V, Pession A, Serra L et al: Non-Hodgkin's lymphoma in children: results of treatment with the modified LSA2-L2 protocol. Med Ped Oncol 1981 (9):483-491
34 Patte C, Kalifa C, Bernard A, Hartmann O, Flamant F, Brugière L, Caillaud JM, Bayle C, Rodary C, Lemerle J: Non-Hodgkin's lymphoma (NHL) in childhood: improvement of survival and CNS prophylaxis in two consecutive studies. Med Ped Oncol 1988 (16):388 (abstract)
35 Patte C, Kalifa C, Bernard A, Hartmann O, Flamant F, Caillaud JM, Bayle C, Lemerle J: LSA2L2 protocol modified by the adjunction of high dose methotrexate (HD MTX): results on 47 children with lymphoblastic non-Hodgkin's lymphomas. Proc of the XVIII Annual Meeting of SIOP, 1986, p 66
36 Biron P, Philip T, Meziane F, Bouffet E, Rebattu P, Frappaz D, Colin C, Brunat-Mentigny M: T lymphoblastic and immunoblastic lymphoma treated with a modification of LSA2L2: 78% relapse-free survival at 36 months. Med Ped Oncol 1988 (16):419 (abstract)
37 Dluzniewska A, Depowska T, Armata J: "Smouldering" and symptomatic forms of central nervous system involvement in the course of non-Hodgkin's lymphoma in children. Folia Haematol Leipzig 1985 (2):241-247
38 Benz-Lemoine E, Leverger G, Bancillon A, Schmitt C, Lamagnere JP, Taboureau O, Perel Y, Schalson G: Treatment of thoracic lymphoblastic lymphoma and acute lymphoblastic leukemia (ALL) with mediastinal mass. Results of "high-risk Fralle 83" protocol in 67 children. Med Ped Oncol 1988 (16):386 (abstract)

Bone Marrow Transplantation for Non-Hodgkin's Lymphoma in Europe: The Current Position

A.H. Goldstone and A.K. McMillan

Department of Haematology, University College Hospital, London WC 1, United Kingdom

The 1989 review of the European bone marrow transplant registry (EBMT) database for Non-Hodgkin's Lymphoma (NHL) reveals that significant numbers of long-term survivors are found after autologous bone marrow transplantation (ABMT) in patient groups in which one might not expect long-term survivors with conventional chemotherapy [1]. This applies to patients who have a good partial remission to first-line chemotherapy and to patients who have relapsed after achieving a complete remission. These results are consistent with the aims of the current policies for patient selection in NHL of the major individual transplant centres. The fundamental question at the present time is whether this contention can be documented in randomised prospective studies. Until this is achieved, the doubt will remain that patient selection has enabled the good results to be achieved. If the role of ABMT in relapse or first partial remission is accepted, then the next question will be whether it is justifiable to transplant any patients in first remission. In this review, we will examine the 1989 EBMT data on ABMT in NHL, describe the randomised studies which are now underway, and then discuss the problem of first remission ABMT. In addition, we will consider for patients with NHL undergoing ABMT, the significance of recombinant human growth factors, conditioning regimens, therapy given after the transplant, and we will compare the results with those of allogeneic BMT.

The 1989 Review of the EBMT Lymphoma Registry

The EBMT data base now receives information from 68 centres throughout Europe and also includes data from three of the largest centres in the USA. In 1989, the data on 698 patients with NHL was analysed, of whom 583 were adults and 115 children. The male:female ratio was 2:1 and the order of frequency of the histologies was high grade, intermediate grade, lymphoblastic and Burkitt's. Patients grafted in first remission account for 28% of the total, but this figure includes a large number of patients with Burkitt's and lymphoblastic lymphoma.

There were 91 deaths during the procedure (13%). However, the interesting fact was that this could be demonstrated to be correlated with the status of the patient at time of transplant. Thus, the figures for first-remission patients (6.7%) and for patients in partial remission (2.6%) can be contrasted with those for responding relapse (18.6%), resistant relapse (15.2%) and primary refractory disease (21.5%). This observation lends weight to the arguments advocating ABMT in first complete remission (1st CR) as the toxicity of the procedure appears to be small for patients in remission.

The overall actuarial disease-free survival for the whole group is approximately 40% at 4 years with a convincing plateau from 2 years onwards. Indeed, the survival curve contrasts with that for Hodgkin's disease in which any plateau is much less likely, due to late relapse occurring beyond 4 years. The NHL survival curve, however, is much more

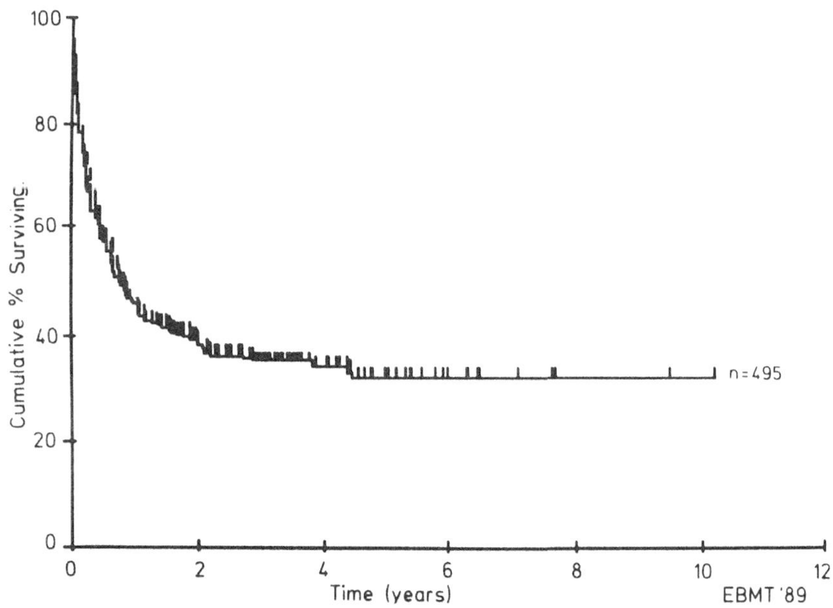

Fig. 1. Overall survival for all patients treated with ABMT in NHL beyond first remission

meaningful if the patients grafted in first remission are excluded, leaving those patients whose prognosis with conventional therapy is very poor (Fig. 1). For this group, the overall actuarial disease-free survival is around 30% with again a plateau beyond 2 years. The tendency to rapid progression in those patients who do not achieve CR is marked with few survivors for any significant time in the patients who do not achieve CR with the graft. Indeed, the exceptions to this are probably due to those patients having non-progressive residual masses rather than an incomplete response to the conditioning regimen.

However, it is notable that when the group who are in CR at the time of the graft are compared with those who achieve CR to the graft, there is no difference in the long-term outcome. This would imply that there is no advantage after relapse to achieving a second CR before a graft. Patients in second remission do no better after a graft than those in responding relapse who are converted to CR by the graft. In addition, one can predict that patients achieving CR in response to the graft have a 50% chance of long-term survival. Once again, the effect of achieving CR

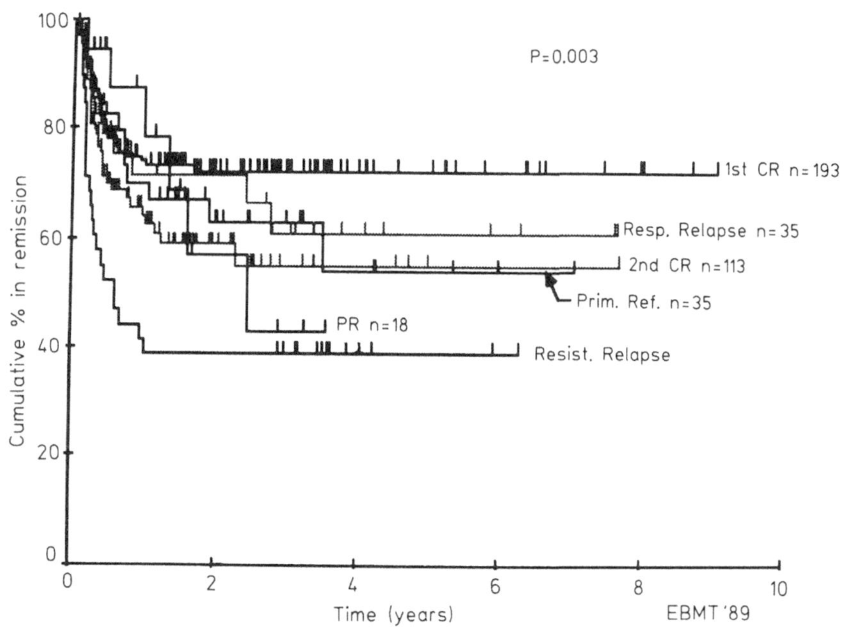

Fig. 2. NHL patients achieving CR at ABMT. Disease-free survival after ABMT by status

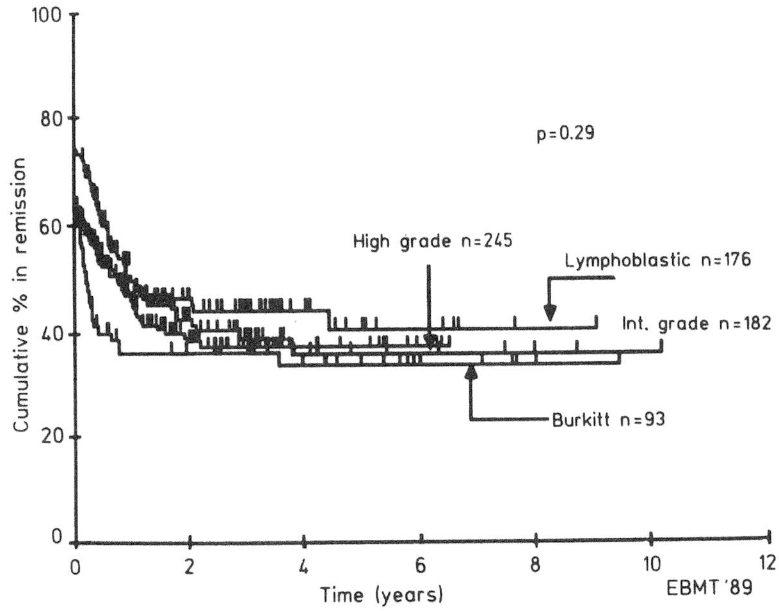

Fig. 3. NHL - Disease-free survival by histology

overrides previously adverse variables (Fig. 2), for example, the data suggests that even those patients with primary refractory disease who do achieve a CR have a disease-free survival of just less than 60%.

Status at time of graft is significantly correlated with disease-free survival both on univariate and on multivariate ($p < 0.0001$) analysis. The chemoresistant group, which comprises patients with resistant relapse and primary refractory disease, has the worst outlook, with an overall disease-free survival of around 20%. Figure 3 shows that overall disease-free survival is similar for all histologies, but on multivariate analysis histology is significantly correlated with disease-free survival ($p < 0.002$). The reason for the apparent contradiction to this finding from that shown in Figure 3 is the tendency in the "worse" histologies to consider ABMT at an earlier stage in the disease. On univariate analysis the stage at diagnosis is not significantly correlated with disease-free survival, which therefore suggests that, at diagnosis, the most important parameter is disease chemosensitivity rather than disease bulk. Mass size at transplantation is significant on univariate analysis in terms of achieving long-term disease-free survival, but not in multivariate analysis; this is most probably because of the close correlation between mass size at ABMT and status at ABMT.

Lastly, we have examined the registry with regard to the efficacy of purging (on multivariate analysis $p = 0.72$) and there is no evidence of any benefit in any of the individual histologies. Our local experience is that around 80% of relapses occur at a site of previous disease, often at sites of bulk disease and this would suggest that, until ablative regimens improve, there is little chance of demonstrating any advantage to purging in the remaining 20%.

Randomised Studies in Progress

As a result of this registry data, the first two prospective randomised studies have emerged (Table 1). The first, labelled "The Parma Study", grew out of discussions originally held at Parma, Italy (Fig. 4), and the second was devised by the British National Lymphoma Investigation (BNLI) following the initial extensive experience at University College and Middlesex Hospital, London (Fig. 5). The Parma study is an International Autologous Bone Marrow Transplant Registry (IABMTR) study.

Table 1. Parma and BNLI chemotherapy protocols

Salvage	Conditioning
Parma study	
DHAP dexamethasone cis-platinum cytarabine	BEAC BCNU etoposide cytarabine cyclophosphamide
BNLI study	
MITOPAC mitozantrone cytarabine prednisolone	BEAM BCNU etoposide cytarabine melphalan
	Mini-BEAM: same drugs as in BEAM but at non-ablative doses

Both studies are aiming to address the problem of whether ABMT can be shown to be of value in a prospective randomised fashion. The Parma study is based on the hypothesis first put forward by Philip et al. [2] that only patients with responding relapse should be autografted. The BNLI study uses a single course of Mitopac chemotherapy to document chemosensitivity, but the response to the salvage chemotherapy, unlike in the Parma study, does not dictate whether an ABMT is performed. The aim of this latter strategy is to document whether the distinction between responding and resistant relapse provides a useful prognostic indicator prospectively in the decision to autograft patients. The BNLI study grafts patients not responding to the salvage regimen (Mitopac) because there is conflicting data as to whether the resistant relapse patients can be salvaged at all. The idea of the mini-BEAM arm is to look at dose escalation using the same drugs with and without transplantation. The EBMT data base does show long-term survival for a small group of resistant relapse patients. The re-

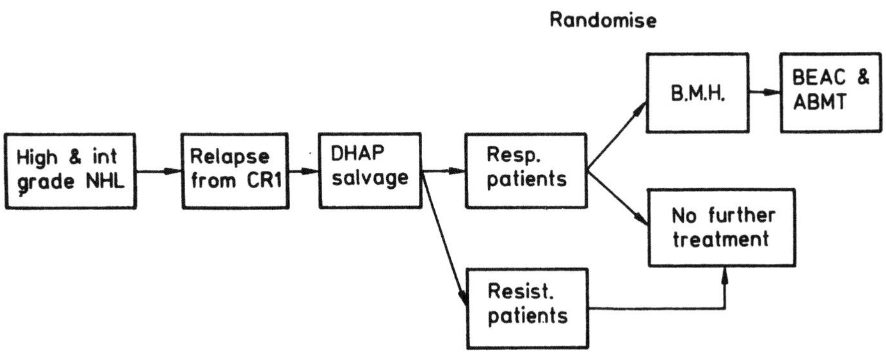

Fig. 4. Parma study

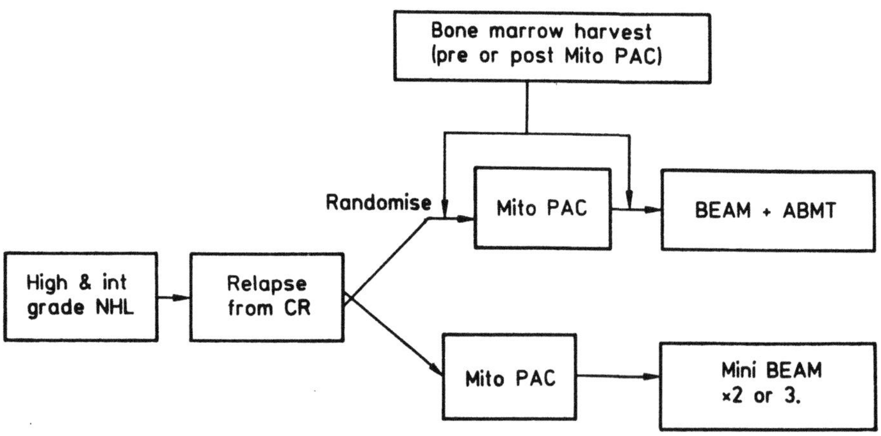

Fig. 5. BNLI study

cruitment of both studies will be critical in determining whether they will be able to produce a meaningful result for, as ABMT becomes more widely publicised, it may become difficult to randomise patients. This is likely to be less of a problem for the BNLI study where the transplant arm is compared with an alternative therapy (Mini-BEAM) as opposed to the Parma study which compares transplantation with no further therapy after a longer salvage regimen.

When is ABMT in First Remission Justified?

The problem with registry data is that no information on the patients *not transplanted* is recorded and therefore conclusions cannot be drawn as to whether the outcome of autografts carried out in first remission are superior to conventional therapy. For example, the overall disease-free survival of 65% in patients autografted in first-remission NHL may either be superior to conventional management if the patients transplanted are genuinely a bad prognostic group or be no different from the best results with conventional therapy if the group is merely a cross-section of the NHL population as a whole. It is also probable that, amongst the 6% procedure-related deaths of grafts performed in first remission, there would be some who were already cured by conventional chemotherapy. Therefore, the disease-free survivals shown in Figure 6 must be compared with the first-remission survivals of these groups without ABMT. This problem is further complicated by the fact that the outcome of non-transplant regimens may be improving due to increasing intensity of therapy, so the transplant results have to be compared with the results of the best current conventional therapies. The BNLI data [3] would suggest that adverse prognostic features at diagnosis are lost if CR is achieved and the EBMT registry data favours this contention, as neither the stage at diagnosis nor the size of the largest mass is significantly correlated with outcome post-graft, whereas both features are significant at time of ABMT in determining outcome. Likewise, previous bone marrow involvement - if cleared by time of grafting - is not a significant prognostic factor. Therefore, it is the current view of the authors that, apart from lymphoblastic lymphoma, which is considered below, there is currently no justification for ABMT in first-remission NHL. The low procedure-related death rate in first CR patients means, however, that a prospective randomised trial of ABMT in first CR for patients with adverse prognostic features at diagnosis would be justified to test this hypothesis, but would be difficult to carry out and would require large numbers of patients to give a meaningful result.

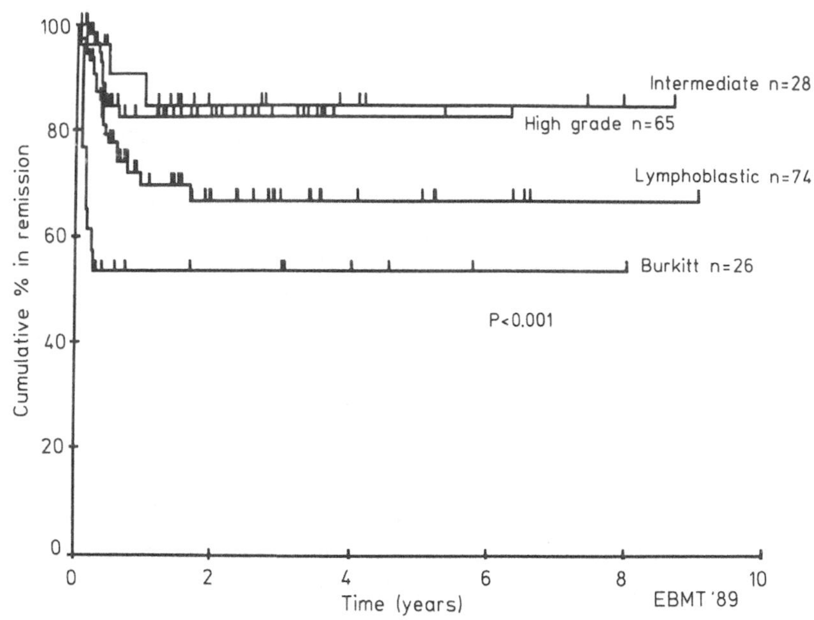

Fig. 6. NHL - ABMT in first CR. Disease-free survival by histology

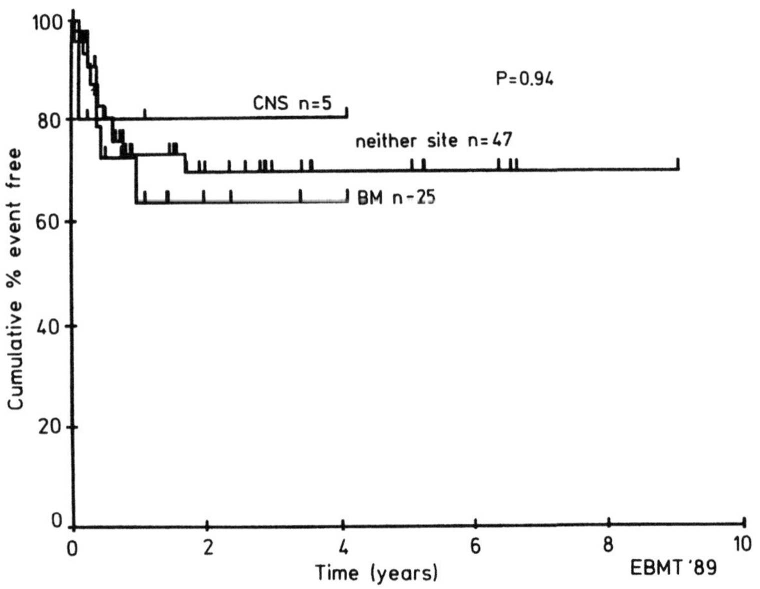

Fig. 7. Lymphoblastic lymphoma - first CR at ABMT. Disease-free survival of those with previous CNS or bone marrow involvement vs the rest

ABMT in First Remission of T-Cell Lymphoblastic Lymphoma

Whether or not to graft in first remission is to be the subject of an EBMT/IABMTR study in patients at high risk of relapse. T-cell lymphoblastic lymphoma (T-LBL) is a highly curable disease for low-risk patients with a projected survival of greater than 90% at 5 years, however, for high-risk patients as defined by Coleman [4] the outlook is much worse, with a projected survival at 5 years of less than 20%. There is clearly no indication for ABMT in the low-risk group, but the high-risk patients represent a suitable group to study whether dose escalation in first remission with autologous or allogeneic bone marrow rescue can improve survival. These patients are those with bone marrow or CNS involvement at diagnosis or a serum LDH of >300 IU/ml at diagnosis (representing disease bulk). The results of a study of high-dose therapy and BMT in first remission T-LBL have been reported by the Italian non-Hodgkin's Lymphoma Cooperative Study Group (NHLCSG) [5] with cyclophosphamide/TBI (autologous marrow) and also by a French multicentre group - Milpied et al. [6] (allogeneic and autologous marrow). These two groups of patients have both given encouraging preliminary results. The EBMT data shows that LBL patients in first remission have a disease-free survival of between 60 and 70% but, more interestingly, this appears to be true of those with bone marrow involvement at diagnosis as well as the patients who by the above criteria would be low risk (Fig. 7).

Therefore, the hypothesis is that BMT can improve the survival of the high-risk patients and this now needs to be tested in a prospective randomised fashion. The major problem of this trial will be to recruit sufficient patients in such a rare tumour for statistical analysis to be fruitful.

When Is an Allogeneic Transplant Indicated in NHL ?

Only 105 allografts in lymphoma have been reported to the EBMT registry and of these 98 were NHL and 7 in HD. Of the NHL group, only the lymphoblastics are enough in number to provide meaningful figures to compare with autologous BMT. Comparison of the autologous and allogeneic (allogeneic lymphoma registry data from Dr. P. Ernst) groups leads to the interesting conclusion that there is no clear indication of any situation in lymphoma where an allogeneic graft with its higher risk and cost can be justified, with the possible exception of second-remission lymphoblastic lymphoma. In particular, there is no advantage of allografting for patients with previous bone marrow involvement. All patients with NHL allografted in relapse do badly. The problem of patients with bone mar

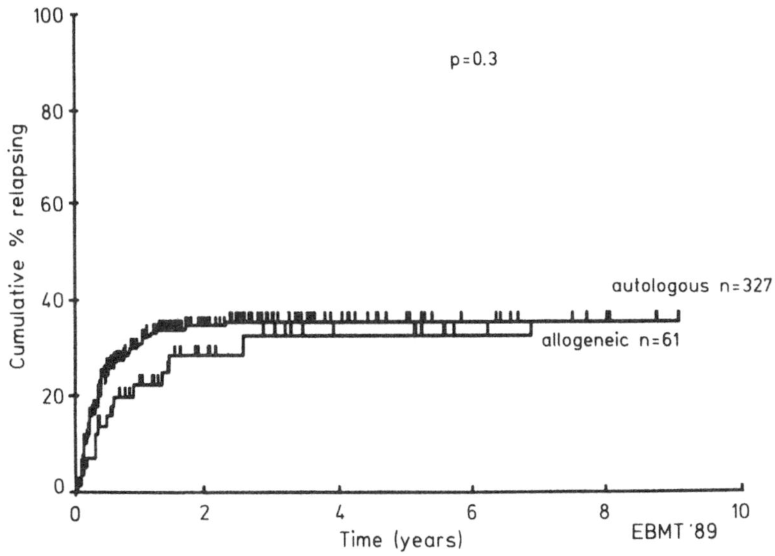

Fig. 8. NHL in remission: probability of relapse for autologous vs allogeneic BMT

row involvement at relapse who cannot be autografted is probably insoluble with present conditioning regimens and cannot be solved by allogeneic transplantation. Our own policy is sometimes to give mini-BEAM to see if the marrow is easily cleared of disease and to then reconsider the patient. Figure 8 shows that there is no difference in the relapse rates between autologous and allogeneic transplantation, thus, there is, on the basis of the registry data, no evidence for a graft-versus-lymphoma effect.

Recombinant Growth Factors and ABMT

This is an area of topical interest but the role of these factors has yet to be clearly defined. The majority of the studies reported dealt with solid tumours [7,8] or with Hodgkin's disease [9,10], but the conclusions from these are likely to be applicable to ABMT in NHL as well. The first growth factor used was granulocyte-macrophage colony-stimulating factor (GM-CSF), which has its main effect at a relatively early stage in myelopoiesis. These studies demonstrated an acceleration of engraftment in the granulocyte series, but the effect on the procedure-related toxicity and the period of hospitalisation was not marked. This may be due to a variety of factors. Firstly, there is no effect on platelet regeneration; secondly, toxicity is often either non-haematological or occurs before leukocyte recovery occurs, even in the growth-factor group. In addition, GM-CSF has a number of effects on mature phagocytes, including, for example, ability impairment of migration response to chemotactic factors [11]. Further trials are now being reported with the more lineage-specific granulocyte colony stimulating factor (G-CSF) and it has been suggested that this factor may be more useful clinically because it does not inhibit the actions of mature phagocytes [11]. Macrophage stimulating factor (M-CSF) is currently under investigation, which, unlike GM-CSF, is non-recombinant, being derived by purification from human urine. Significant reductions in the period of hospitalisation, which is mainly dictated by platelet recovery, may have to await the isolation of thrombopoietin or the use of combinations of growth factors to achieve the same effect.

Further Therapy Post-Graft

Many centres advocate the use of consolidation radiotherapy to sites of bulk disease following autografts with high-dose chemotherapy. This is a rational approach based on the observation that most relapses occur at sites of bulk disease [12] and the dire prognosis of relapse post-graft. At our centre we have applied this policy in a group of Hodgkin's disease autografts without seeing significant toxicity when the radiation is given at 3 months post-graft [13]. A multicentre trial would be unlikely to accrue patients because individual centres would wish to irradiate particular patients, therefore, the establishment of the efficacy of this radiation is likely to be impossible. It is likely to continue but without a proven basis, though this probably does not matter as long as it is genuinely without significant toxicity. The rationale to irradiate sites of previous bulk disease may be less strong in NHL, in which relapse is more likely to be at new sites than is the case for Hodgkin's disease.

The second form of post-graft therapy to be considered is immune modulation, using cytokines such as interleukins or interferons. The use of these agents is most likely to be valuable when a state of minimal residual disease has been achieved, but until toxicity studies have been performed the commencement of the large trials necessary to document efficacy will be delayed. The results in advanced lymphoma are not encouraging [14] and until immune modulators have been shown to work in this situation and the basic concept of autografting has been established in multicentre trials, it is inappropriate to commence trials of cytokines in ABMT, except to study toxicity. Compliance with such therapy both by physicians in the referral centres and by the patients who perceive ABMT as a single intensive therapy may not be good with this type of study.

Conditioning Regimens

The EBMT database does not show any advantage for total body irradiation (TBI) regimens over chemotherapy ablation. TBI probably is more toxic and is not advised if the chest or mediastinum have been irradiated. The various chemotherapy regimens, such as BEAM, BEAC and CBV, are comprised of similar drugs and appear to be yielding similar results. In addition, ablation with chemotherapy makes the use of local irradiation post-graft a feasibility. Unless new data can disprove it, the hypothesis that all high-dose regimens yield similar results seems sound at present.

Conclusions

The time has come for randomised clinical trials to document the efficacy of autografting in lymphoma. All patients should be considered for one of the national or international trials that are open. The view in many parts of the United States that autografting is already proven to be of value is not tenable at present, and the proponents of ABMT must be patient and await the proof of their opinions. The use of growth factors may be an advance, but this is also unproven at present. The gradual improvement of conventional therapy of NHL and the use of growth factors to facilitate intensive dosage in this situation must be remembered when assessing patients for ABMT. Apart from lymphoblastic lymphoma, there seems little justification for first-remission ABMT.

REFERENCES

1 Goldstone AH, Gribben JG, McMillan AK, Taghipour G: The sixth report of the EBMTG Registry of ABMT in Lymphoma. Proceedings of the XVth meeting of the EBMT (1989). BMT suppl (in press)

2 Philip T, Armitage JO, Spitzer G, Chauvin F, Jagganath S, Cahn J-Y, Colombat P, Goldstone AH, Gorin NC, Flesh M, Laporte J-P, Maraninchi D, Pico J, Bosly J, Anderson C, Schuts R, Biron P, Cabinillas F, Dicke K: High dose therapy and ABMT after failure of conventional therapy in adults with intermediate grade or high grade non-Hodgkin's lymphoma. N Engl J Med 1987 (316):1493-1498

3 Linch DC and Vaughan-Hudson B: The management of Hodgkin's disease and the non-Hodgkin's lymphomas. In: Hoffbrand AV (ed) Recent Advances in Haematology V. Churchill Livingstone, London 1988 pp 211-242

4 Coleman CN, Picozzi VJ, Cox RS, McWhirter K, Weiss LM, Cohen JR, Yu KP, Rosenberg SA: Treatment of lymphoblastic lymphoma in adults. J Clin Oncol 1987 (4):1628-1637

5 Santini G, Coser P, Rizzoli P, Congiu AM, Chisesi T, Sertoli R, Porcellini A, Contu A, Rossi E, Carella A, Scarpati D, Raffo MR, Nati S, Gaozza E, Marmont AM: ABMT in advanced stages of adult lymphoblastic lymphoma (LBL) in first CR. A report of the NHLCSG (Italy).BMT 1988 (3 suppl 1):297

6 Milpied N, Ifrah N, Kuentz M, Maraninchi D, Colombat P, Harousseau JL: Bone marrow transplantation for adult poor prognosis lymphoblastic lymphoma in first complete remission. BMT 1988 (3 suppl 1):63

7 Brandt SJ, Peters WP, Atwater S, Kurtzburg J, Borowitz MJ, Jones RB, Shpall EJ, Bast RC, Gilbert CJ, Oette DH: Effect of recombinant human granulocyte-macrophage colony-stimulating factor on haematopoietic reconstitution after high dose chemotherapy and autologous bone marrow transplantation. N Engl J Med 1988 (318):869-875

8 Antman KS, Griffin JD, Ellias A, Socinski A, Ryan L, Cannistra SA, Oette D, Whitley M, Frei E, Schnipper LE: Effect of recombinant human granulocyte-macrophage colony-stimulating factor on chemotherapy-induced myelosuppression. N Engl J Med 1989 (319):593-598

9 Devereux S, Linch DC, Gribben JG, McMillan AK, Patterson K, Goldstone AH: GM-CSF accelerates neutrophil recovery after autologous bone marrow transplantation. BMT 1989 (4):49-54

10 Taylor K, Spitzer g, Jagganath S, Dicke K, Souza L: Phase II study of recombinant human granulocyte colony-stimulating factor in Hodgkin's disease after high dose chemotherapy with ABMT. Blood 1988 (5 suppl 1):452

11 Peters WP, Kurtzburg J, Atwater S, Borowitz M, Gilbert C,, Rao M, Currie M, Shogan J, Jones RB, Shpall EJ, Souza L: Comparitive effects of rHuG-CSF and rHuGM-CSF on haematopoietic reconstitution and granulocyte function following high dose chemotherapy and autologous bone marrow transplantation. Blood 1988 (5 suppl 1):432

12 Goldstone AH, Linch DC, Gribben JG, McMillan AK: Experience of autologous bone marrow transplantation in the first 100 lymphomas. BMT 1988 (3 suppl 1):65

13 McMillan AK, Tobias JS, Gribben JG, Linch DC & Goldstone AH: Radiotherapy for residual Hodgkin's disease after BEAM chemotherapy and autologous bone marrow transplantation. Proceedings of the XVth meeting of the EBMT (1989). BMT suppl (in press)

14 Duggan D, Anderson J,Zamkoff K, Poiesz B, Ozer H, Bloomfield C, Gottlieb A, Syracuse NY, Brookline MA: Interleukin 2 alone or with b-Interferon in relapsed non-Hodgkin's lymphoma - Preliminary report of CALGB 8653. Blood 1988 (5 suppl 1):876

Non-Hodgkin's Lymphomas in Patients with AIDS

U. Tirelli, E. Vaccher, D. Errante, I. Crosato, G. Rezza, A. Lazzarin, R. Foà, S. Pileri, A. Carbone, G. Ambrosini, A. Andriani, M. Barberis, M. Barbui, C. Bernasconi, I. Bianco Silvestroni, A. Borri, G. Bottinelli, G. Broccia, P.L. Bullian, A. Cajozzo, A. Cargnel, P. Cazzaniga, F. Chiodo, T. Chisesi, M. Clerici, P. Costigliola, P. Crocchiolo, F. De Lalla, M. Della Santa, P. Dessalvi, F. Fiaccadori, F. Figoli, M. Fiorentino, M. Franchi, P.L. Garavelli, F. Gherlinzoni, F. Gianelli, M.G. Giudici, C. Guglielmi, G. Lambertenghi Deliliers, F. Lanza, F. Lombardi, G. Luzi, R. Luzzati, A. Malfitano, C. Malleo, F. Mandelli, M. Marangolo, A. Maringos, G. Martignoni, D. Milo, V. Montesarchio, L. Ortona, G. Palmieri, E.A. Parrinello, N. Piersantelli, G. Pizzoccaro, C, Pristerà, F. Puppo, A. Quaglino, E. Raise, A. Riccardi, E. Ricchi, G. Rizzardini, M. Rizzi, F. Rizzo, A.M. Rosci, G. Rossi, S. Sabbatani, G. Saliva, G. Salvi, S. Saracchini, G. Scalise, A. Scanni, A. Sinicco, R. Sorio, V.A. Squadrini, R. Stellini, V. Stracca Pansa, E. Sulis, A. Surbone, A. Terragna, A. Tognetti, A. Vaglia, R. Zagni, V. Zagonel, F. Gavosto, S. Monfardini

Italian Cooperative Group for AIDS-related Tumours

The increased incidence of malignancies associated with AIDS has been the subject of several reports in the North American literature: besides Kaposi's sarcoma and other tumours, such as squamous carcinoma of the tongue and cloacogenic carcinoma of the anorectum [1-22], malignant lymphomas have been demonstrated to be one of the major problems among the neoplastic complications of AIDS [12-24]. According to the North American experience, non-Hodgkin's lymphomas in patients with AIDS or AIDS-related clinical conditions present at an advanced stage in which lesions are concentrated in extranodal and often unusual locations, notably the CNS. Disease confined to the lymph nodes is uncommon. These lymphomas are predominantly high-grade B-cell neoplasms classified as immunoblastic and Burkitt's-like lymphomas. A variety of severe opportunistic infections and Kaposi's sarcoma affect these patients. At the same time, the association with AIDS is strengthened by the regular demonstration of reversed ratios of helper (T4+) and suppressor (T8+) lymphocytes in the peripheral blood and by the presence of antibodies to human immune deficiency virus (HIV) [22]. The prognosis is dismal: response to chemotherapy does not positively affect median survival. Mortality rates analysed by histological grade are higher than the currently reported rates for comparable patient populations [18].

The majority of cases of malignant lymphomas in patients in the United States at risk of, or with AIDS, have been reported in homosexuals, leading to the conclusion that malignant lymphomas in this risk group are more common than in other high-risk patients, such as i.v. drug abusers (IVDA) [22].

At present, not much information on the neoplastic complications of AIDS in Europe is available, but medical oncologists and haematologists are aware, from personal experience or contact with colleagues, that such cases are beginning to be observed among the countries of the European Economic Community. So far, only one report dealing with the pathological characteristics of malignant lymphomas in patients with AIDS has been published in France [25], and only sporadic cases have been reported in other countries of the EEC [26-29].

For these reasons, this report, a survey by an Italian Cooperative Group on the incidence and clinicopathological characteristics of malignant lymphomas in patients with AIDS or at risk for AIDS in Italy, may help bring the present situation in Europe into better focus.

Patients and Methods

At the Centro Oncologico of Aviano and at the Clinica Medica I of the University of Turin, the Italian Cooperative Group on AIDS-related Tumours (GICAT) was organised in November 1986, with the aim of looking at the incidence and outcome of malignant lymphomas in persons with AIDS or at high risk for AIDS in Italy.

A total of 1,962 questionnaires were sent to members of the Italian Societies for Medical Oncology, Haematology and Immunology and to selected infectious disease specialists. These investigators, at each of the participating institutions, were asked to identify all known patients at risk for AIDS (homosexuals, IVDA, haemophiliacs, polytransfused persons) in whom a malignant lymphoma (non-Hodgkin's lymphoma or Hodgkin's disease) had developed between January 1980 and November 1987. Concurrently, the same information on HIV infection-related lymphomas was obtained from the Italian Ministry of Health for all reported cases of AIDS in Italy. A revised and integrated form was then sent to investigators who had previously reported cases of malignant lymphomas (42 centres) to better specify information about initial localisation, histological subtype, clinical stage, treatment response, toxicity, development of AIDS-associated conditions, and survival from time of treatment to death or to November 1987. This evaluation was carried out only on the basis of the data collected through the initial and then integrated questionnaires and through case-by-case discussion with the medical staff responsible in each centre for each patient, but without pathology review of the material. The criteria used to diagnose persistent generalised lymphadenopathy (PGL) and AIDS were conform to those established by the Centre for Disease Control (CDC) [30]. HIV serology was performed by enzyme-linked immunosorbent assay and reconfirmed by Western blot (immunoblot). Actuarial survival was determined by the method of Kaplan and Meier [31].

Results

By November 1987, 95 cases of non-Hodgkin's lymphomas had been reported from different centres in Italy. One patient was observed before 1983, while most cases were observed at an increasing rate after 1984. In particular, 5 patients were observed in 1984, 19 in 1985, 48 in 1986, and 57 in 1987. Not all data, including those on follow up, were generally available in all cases, due to the peculiar features of this population of patients, such as frequent change of address and of physician and other economic and logistical problems connected with i.v. drug abuse.

Table 1 shows the currently available information on persons with AIDS or at risk for AIDS and with non-Hodgkin's lymphoma in Italy. In each of the clinicopathological characteristics reported in this Table and discussed below, the denominator refers to the number of patients for whom the information was available. The patients were predominantly male (79%). Most of the patients with non-Hodgkin's lymphoma had AIDS, while only a small number presented with PGL or AIDS-related complex (ARC), using the CDC criteria for a diagnosis of AIDS, PGL, or ARC. Three patients at risk (1 polytransfused, 1 IVDA and 1 homosexual) were HIV negative. Overall, there were more IVDA than homosexuals, polytransfused persons and haemophiliacs. The median age was 27 years. High-grade histology was present in 70 out of 81 patients (86%), with a consistent percentage of patients with high-grade histology showing Burkitt's-like histology (37%). Among 67 patients for whom information on initial presentation was available, extranodal disease at onset was present in 61. Initial sites in these 67 patients were: CNS, 25 cases (37%); bone marrow, 18 (27%); liver, 24 (36%); spleen, 17 (25%); stomach, 10 (15%); small bowel, 2 (3%); skin, 6 (9%);

Table 1. Non-Hodgkin's lymphomas in persons at risk for or with AIDS in Italy

Characteristics	No. of patients/No. included	(%)*
Sex		
Male	70/95	(79)
Female	20/95	(21)
Median age in yrs (range): 27 (19-64)		
HIV seropositive	89/92 **	(97)
Diagnosis		
PGL	5/91	(5)
AIDS	85/91	(93)
ARC	0/91	
HIV seropositive	1/91	(1)
Risk group		
IVDA	63/93	(68)
Homosexual	17/93	(18)
IVDA + homosexual	5/93	(5)
Heterosexual	3/93	(3)
Polytransfused	2/93	(2)
Unknown	2/93	(2)
Haemophiliac	1/93	(1)
Histological grade		
Low	4/81	(5)
Intermediate	7/81	(9)
High	70/81	(86)
Burkitt's-like	16/43	(37)
Stage		
I	2/75	(3)
I, extranodal involvement***	21/75	(28)
II	3/75	(4)
III	4/75	(5)
IV	45/75	(60)

* No. included = number for whom data were available (total number = 95)
** 3 patients at risk were HIV seronegative
*** 19 CNS, 1 lung, 1 gastrointestinal tract

lung, 6 (9%); kidney, 4 (6%); pancreas, 2 (3%); ovary, 1 (1%); larynx, 1 (1%); adrenal gland 1 (1%); and nasopharynx, 1 (1%). No primary sites, oral or anorectal localisations concomitant with other sites of disease were observed. Opportunistic infections at onset were present in 47% of patients (34 out of 72 evaluable patients). The median latency between PGL and the appearance of the malignant lymphoma was 14 months.

Half of the patients for whom information on therapy was available (34 out of 68 patients) could not receive any antineoplastic therapy because of either rapid disease progression, treatment refusal, death, or postmortem diagnosis. Twenty-three patients received various combination chemotherapy regimens (cyclophosphamide, vincristine and prednisone; cyclophosphamide, doxorubicin, vincristine and prednisone; doxorubicin, cyclophosphamide, methotrexate, prednisone and etoposide (ProMACE); mechlorethamine, vincristine, procarbazine and prednisone (MOPP); ProMACE/cytarabine, bleomycin, vincristine and methotrexate, and others), and 3 patients received combination chemotherapy and radiotherapy, but only 9 out of 26 (35%) patients achieved complete remission (CR) and 12 out of 26 (46%) achieved partial remission (PR). Of 7 patients (for whom clini

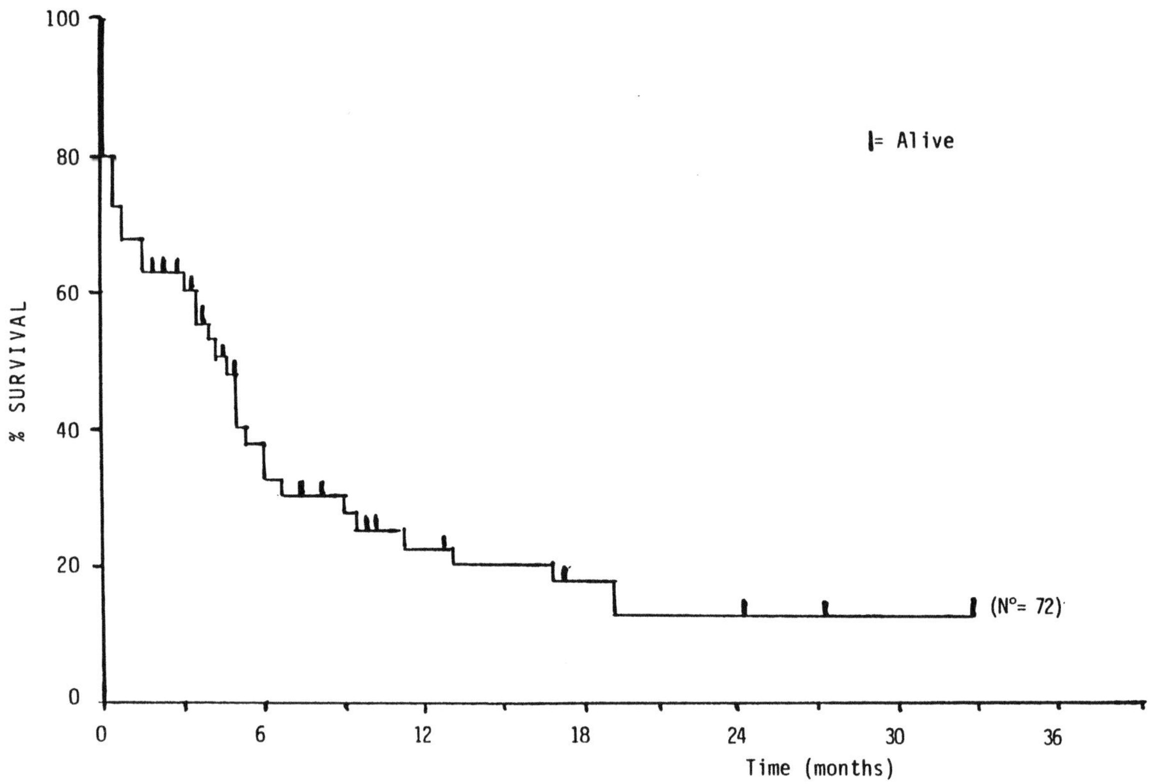

Fig. 1. Overall survival: non-Hodgkin's lymphomas-AIDS (N=72 patients)

cal information was available) achieving CR, only 1 presented initially with opportunistic infection, while 5 presented with PGL and 1 was HIV seropositive only. As of November 1987, 53 out of 72 (74%) patients were dead. As the cause of death, progression of the disease accounted for 26 deaths (49%), 11 patients died of opportunistic infections, 4 of tumour progression and opportunistic infections, 2 of internal haemorrhage, 2 of disseminated intravascular coagulation, 1 of acute renal failure, 1 of hepatic toxicity, and 6 of unknown causes. The median survival of patients with non-Hodgkin's lymphomas was only 4 months (Fig. 1).

With regard to the 3 patients who were in the AIDS risk group but HIV negative, with high-grade non-Hodgkin's lymphoma, the disease progressed rapidly, as it did in other patients who were HIV positive. Kaposi's sarcoma was associated with non-Hodgkin's lymphomas in only 1 patient.

Discussion

Non-Hodgkin's lymphoma of Burkitt's type is one of the earliest recognised manifestations of AIDS [18]. According to the CDC definition [32], non-Hodgkin's lymphomas of high-grade histology or of CNS origin occurring in HIV-seropositive patients are diagnostic of AIDS, even in the absence of opportunistic infections or Kaposi's sarcoma. Six large series of AIDS-related non-Hodgkin's lymphoma cases [12,15,18-21] have been reported from the United States. Non-Hodgkin's lymphomas present extranodal involvement and are correlated with a short survival. Recently, the pathological characteristics of 21 cases of non-Hodgkin's lymphomas associated with AIDS have been described in Paris, while so far only sporadic cases have been reported in the rest of Europe [25-29].

This report suffers from the obvious limitation of being a retrospective cooperative study on a problem the importance of which has only recently emerged, but not necessarily at a time when clinical observations could be made. However, this study is the result of the only nationwide inquiry conducted in Europe and to our knowledge is the largest IVDA-based case series ever reported in the English literature.

These data reveal for the first time the presence in Italy of a consistent number of malignant lymphomas among persons with HIV infections or at risk for AIDS (4 patients). Although preliminary, this information confirms that patients with non-Hodgkin's lymphomas have an increased incidence of high-grade subtypes, particularly in Burkitt's type, present at an advanced stage with frequent extranodal involvement, and have a short median survival. Most of the cases of non-Hodgkin's lymphomas were observed in IVDA; however, the clinicopathological characteristics of these AIDS-associated cases were, in general, comparable to those reported in North American case series, in which homosexuals predominated. However, we did not observe primary oral or anorectal lymphomas, or involvement of the oral and anorectal area during the course of non-Hodgkin's lymphoma, as reported in the United States by several authors [18,22-24]. This might be the result of the small number of homosexuals in our series in whom these manifestations were described.

The prevalence of AIDS-associated non-Hodgkin's lymphomas among IVDA in Italy was in agreement with the overall incidence of AIDS, which is 59% for IVDA, 22% for homosexuals, 4.2% for homosexual IVDA, 4.8% for haemophiliacs and polytransfused persons, and 2.8% for heterosexuals out of the 1,200 cases reported as of August 1987 [32]. In the United States, the reported incidence of AIDS is much higher for homosexuals (65%) and lower for IVDA (16%) [33]. From the analysis of accumulated case series in this country [12-21] of AIDS-associated non-Hodgkin's lymphomas, 89% were reported among homosexuals and 10% among IVDA; in New York City, however, although AIDS-related non-Hodgkin's lymphomas were reported mainly among homosexual men, 30% of overall AIDS cases occurred among IVDA [12,33]. It can be deduced that in both countries the different occurrence of AIDS-associated non-Hodgkin's lymphoma among homosexuals and IVDA reflects the overall spread of the AIDS epidemic among risk groups.

In most patients, PGL was associated with and preceded the development of malignant lymphoma. In fact, some patients presenting with PGL were referred to some of the oncological centres participating in the cooperative study because of the clinical diagnosis of lymphoma. The initial clinical presentation of PGL is similar to that of malignant lymphoma, often being accompanied by malaise, fever, night sweats, weight loss, and splenomegaly [39]. The potential diagnosis of malignant lymphoma should, therefore, be considered for a patient with PGL. More than one biopsy site may be necessary in the investigation of these patients. As time passes and clinical conditions may arouse clinical suspicion of a lymphoma, repeated biopsies may be required.

In conclusion, the problem of AIDS-related tumours deserved attention not only from a clinical point of view, but also in consideration of the possible progress that may be achieved in understanding the aetiology and pathogenesis of the neoplastic complications of AIDS. This report shows that a relatively large number of cases are presently available in Italy, allowing a better study of the virological, immunological, pathological and clinical aspects of the problem. However, epidemiological study remains the key point to detect whether the higher incidence of malignant lymphomas among IVDA than among homosexuals in Italy is entirely attributable to the characteristics of the AIDS epidemic among IVDA in this country or whether other causes may also be responsible for this phenomenon. The need for a registry for the careful collection of data on Italian and other European patients with HIV infection and malignant lymphomas and also for other tumours should receive priority attention.

Acknowledgement

This study was supported by a grant of the "Associazione Italiana per la Ricerca sul Cancro", contract No. 1004:700:86.

REFERENCES

1 Safai B, Koziner B: Malignant neoplasms in AIDS. In: De Vita VT Jr, Hellmann S, Rosenberg SA (eds) AIDS - Etiology, Diagnosis, Treatment and Prevention. Lippincott, Philadelphia 1985 pp 213-222
2 Biggar RJ, Horm J, Lubin JH et al: Cancer trends in a population at risk of acquired immune-deficiency syndrome. JNCI 1985 (4):793-794
3 Hymes KB, Green JB, Marcus A et al: Kaposi sarcoma in homosexual men - a report of eight cases. Lancet 1981 (2):598-600
4 Centers of Disease Control Task Force on Kaposi's Sarcoma and Opportunistic Infections. Epidemiologic aspects of the current outbreak of Kaposi's sarcoma and opportunistic infections. N Engl J Med 1982 (306):248-252
5 Gottlieb GJ, Ragaz A, Vogel JV et al: A preliminary communication on extensively disseminated Kaposi's sarcoma in young homosexual men. Am J Dermatopathol 1981 (3):111-114
6 Safai B: Kaposi's sarcoma and other neoplasms in acquired immunodeficiency syndrome. In: Galin JI, Fauci AS (eds) Advances in Host Defense Mechanisms. Raven Press, New York 1985 pp 59-73
7 Myskowsky PL, Romano JF, Safai B: Kaposi's sarcoma in young homosexual men. Cutis 1983 (29):31-34
8 Friedman-Kien AE, Laubenstein LJ, Raubenstein P et al: Disseminated Kaposi's sarcoma in homosexual men. Ann Intern Med 1982 (96):693-697
9 Groopman JE: Neoplasms in the acquired immunodeficiency syndrome: the multidisciplinary approach to treatment. Semin Oncol 1987 (14 suppl 3):1-6
10 Peters RK, Mack TM: Patterns of anal carcinoma by gender and marital status in Los Angeles County. Br J Cancer 1983 (48):629-636
11 Cooper MS, Patchefsky AS, Marks G: Cloacogenic carcinoma of the anorectum in homosexual men: an observation of four cases. Dis Colon Rectum 1979 (2):557
12 Ahmed T, Wormser GP, Stahl RE et al: Malignant lymphomas in a population at risk for acquired immunodeficiency syndrome. Cancer 1987 (60):719-723
13 Ziegler JL, Miner RC, Rosenbaum E et al: Outbreak of Burkitt's lymphoma in homosexual men. Lancet 1982 (2):631-633
14 Diffuse undifferentiated non-Hodgkin's lymphoma among homosexual males in the United States. Morbid Mortal Weekly Rep 1982:277-279
15 Ioachim HL, Hellmann GC: Lymphomas associated with the acquired immunodeficiency syndrome (AIDS): a study of 35 cases. Cancer Detect Prev 1987 (suppl 1):557-565
16 Jaffe ES, Clark J, Steis R et al: Lymph node pathology of HTLV-associated neoplasm. Cancer Res 1985 (45, suppl):4662S-4664S
17 Shoeppel S, Hoppe R, Abrams D et al: Hodgkin's disease (HD) in homosexual men: the San Francisco Bay Area experience. Presented at the Annual Meeting of the American Society of Clinical Oncology. Houston TX, 1986
18 Ziegler JL, Beckstead AJ, Volberding PA et al: Non-Hodgkin's lymphoma in 90 homosexual men. N Engl J Med 1984 (311):565-570
19 Gill P, Levine AM, Rarick M et al: Malignant non-Hodgkin's lymphomas (NHL) in patients with HIV infection. Presented at the Third International Conference on Malignant Lymphoma. Lugano, Switzerland, 1987
20 Knowles DM, Chamulak G, Subar M et al: Clinical, morphologic, phenotypic and molecular genetic analysis of AIDS/ARC-associated malignant lymphoid neoplasia. Presented at the Third International Conference on Malignant Lymphoma. Lugano, Switzerland, 1987
21 Kaplan LD, Volberding PA, Abrams DI: Update on AIDS-associated non-Hodgkin's lymphoma (NHL) in San Francisco. Presented at the Third International Conference on AIDS. Washington DC, 1987
22 Levine AM: Non-Hodgkin's lymphomas and other malignancies in the acquired immune-deficiency syndrome. Semin Oncol 1987 (14 suppl 3):34-39
23 Ioachim HL, Weinstein MA, Robbins RD et al: Primary anorectal lymphoma. A new manifestation of the acquired immune deficiency syndrome (AIDS). Cancer 1987 (60):1449-1453
24 Burkes RL, Meyer PR, Gill PS et al: Rectal lymphoma in homosexual men. Arch Intern Med 1986 (146):913-915
25 Raphael M, Tulliez M, Bellefoth S et al: Les lymphomes et le SIDA. Ann Pathol 1986 (6):278-281
26 Lev HJ, Schneider J, Hardmeier T et al: Kaposi's sarcoma and malignant lymphoma in AIDS. Virchows Arch 1984 (403):205-212
27 Payan MJ, Gambarelli D, Routy JP et al: Primary lymphoma of the brain associated with AIDS. Acta Neuropathol, Berlin 1984 (64):78-80
28 Casadei GP, Gambacorta M: A clinico-pathological study of seven cases of primary high-grade malignant non-Hodgkin's lymphoma of the central nervous system. Tumori 1985 (71):501-507
29 Skinhoj P, Ersboll J, Nissen NI: Human immunodeficiency virus (HIV) associated non-Hodgkin's lymphomas in Denmark: report of three cases. Eur J Haematol 1987 (39):71-74
30 Anonymous: Case definition of AIDS revised. Morbid Mortal Weekly Rep 1985 (34):373-375
31 Kaplan EL, Meier P: Nonparametric estimation from incomplete observations. J Am Stat Assoc 1958 (53):457-481
32 Anonymous: Aggiornamento sull'AIDS al 30.8.87. Boll Epidemiol Naz 1987 (9):1-5
33 Anonymous: Update: acquired immunodeficiency syndrome - United States. Morbid Mortal Weekly Rep 1987 (36):522-525
34 Zagonel V, Tirelli U, Vaccher E et al: Clinical and laboratory findings at presentation in Persistent Generalized Lymphadenopathy vs Malignant Lymphoma. Cancer Detect Prevent 1988 (12):225-229

Conclusions

S. Monfardini [1], B. Coiffier [2], J. Estapé [3] and G. Gahrton [4]

1 Division of Medical Oncology, Centro di Riferimento Oncologico, Aviano, Italy
2 Haematology Service, Centre Hospitalier Lyon-Sud Pierre Bénite, Lyon, France
3 Oncology Service, Hospital Clinic, Barcelona, Spain
4 Division of Clinical Haematology and Oncology, Department of Medicine, Karolinska Institute at Huddinge Hospital, Huddinge, Sweden

The evaluation of the management of NHL in Europe shows that many European groups are today in the favourable position of carrying out clinical research competitive with that of the North-American Study Groups with respect to number of patients, skill of clinical oncologists and available technologies.

Interpretation of Results

The experience arising from these meetings confirms once more that the basis for future clinical trials is a correct interpretation of previous trials [1]. In particular, the following recommendations can be given for the interpretation of results in unfavourable advanced NHL:

1) Appropriate and accurate diagnosis is essential to assure comparability of trials in NHL. Unfortunately, there is usually a high discordance rate between pathologists: even when highly experienced pathologists are tested for consistency in their diagnosis, the rate of reproducibility may range from 50 to 90% [2]. In recent years, a wider use of immunophenotyping and cytogenetic analysis has improved the definition of many lymphomas of B- and T-cell origin. For the future, the molecular analysis of immunoglobulin gene rearrangement could be a promising tool. The greater precision in the cytohistological identification and the immunological characterisation of NHL has been of help in ensuring more accurate diagnosis, but at the same time has led to new clinicopathological entities not yet included in current NHL lymphoma classifications [3]. For example, lymphomas of the mucose-associated lymphoid tissues (MALT), monocytoid B-cell lymphoma and large anaplastic (K-1) positive lymphoma carry their own prognostic significance and are probably differently represented in the various case series. Peripheral T-cell lymphomas bear a worse prognosis than B-cell lymphomas, independently of all other adverse prognostic factors, and the percentage of patients with either phenotype should be taken into account [4].
2) The most important obstacle to the comparison among studies is the variability of prognostic factors in different populations of patients. The superiority of a new treatment can only be demonstrated if the control group is comparable according to clinical, biological and immunological factors of prognostic value. The clinical factors that appear to be accompanied by a poor prognosis are tumour bulk, low performance status, systemic symptoms, elevated serum LDH and bone marrow involvement. The influence of age is well known and most evident after 70 years. In trials related to elderly patients, not only should the median age be clearly stated, but also how many patients are older than 65 and 70 years.
3) Long-term follow up in comparing regimens is important. CR rates of 60-80%

have been observed with modern intensive combination chemotherapy [5,8], and the relapse rate has decreased. Thus, 50-70% of patients survive 3 years or longer. However, long-term results (5 or 10 years of follow up) are not available for all the new intensive regimens, and thus the advantage in terms of survival is not definitely known. Results with newer regimens require confirmation.

4) "Newer regimens", with more intensive chemotherapy without bone marrow rescue, are at present not likely to add any advantage. Before we have the results of the several ongoing trials prospectively comparing CHOP with more intensive combination chemotherapy such as ProMACE-MOPP, ProMACE-CytaBOM, MACOP-B, new regimens are probably not needed. The escalation of one or more drugs (no new valuable drugs are presently available) of current front-line programmes results in an automatic decrease in the deliverable dose of other active drugs.
5) The efficacy of a treatment regimen including autologous (ABMT) or allogeneic bone marrow transplantation (BMT) should be analysed, taking into account the status of the patient at the time of the transplant (first remission, partial remission, responding relapse, resistant relapse, primary refractory disease), since the initial status is significantly correlated with survival.

Current Treatment Strategies and Possible Recommendations

Follicular Low-Grade NHL

In limited disease (stages I and II), radiotherapy alone on involved fields or involved plus adjacent lymph-node regions is an adequate treatment. Adjuvant chemotherapy may improve the disease-free interval but not overall survival.

In advanced (stage III and IV) low grade NHL it is difficult to give clearcut recommendations since the following roughly equivalent possibilities are available:

1) treatment delay until progression;
2) single-agent chemotherapy with alkylating agents (chlorambucil);
3) combination chemotherapy with CVP or CHOP;
4) total body irradiation (TBI) seems to have lost favour in Europe over the last five years.

Novel strategies in follicular low-grade NHL are intensive chemotherapy with ProMACE-MOPP, high-dose cyclophosphamide and TBI with ABMT in second or subsequent remission. Interferon has been shown to be effective in the treatment of low-grade NHL.

Thus, the questions which future studies should try to answer are:

1) Is there a group of patients in whom treatment could be delayed until progression?
2) Is the dose-response positive relationship also applicable to low-grade NHL?
3) What role can be played by intensification of therapy with bone marrow rescue?
4) How can the novel mechanism of action of Interferon be exploited?

The questions are posed to underline once more that optimal treatment is not known and should be sought by means of large cooperative trials.

High-Grade and Intermediate NHL

Third-generation regimens such as M-BACOP, ProMACE-MOPP, LNH 84 [5,6,7] in centroblastic and immunoblastic NHL have been associated with CR in 60-80% of the patients, with 50-70% surviving 3 years or longer. However, similar long-term survival has been observed in patients of less than 55 years treated with CHOP. Thus, since it is still not clear whether third-generation regimens improve survival compared to the conventional CHOP treatment, the choice of intensive last-generation regimens outside of the context of controlled clinical trials should take into consideration prognostic factors related both to treatment tolerance (age, PS, vital organ function tests) and to the disease (negative prognostic disease factors are bulky disease, more than 3 sites involved, elevated LDH). These factors have been condensed in prognostic indexes that divide pa-

tients in 3 groups of good, intermediate, and bad prognosis [10].
For these histological subgroups ABMT or BMT may well be a choice. At the present time it can be recommended in second remission and at partial remission, but data are still insufficient to recommend these methods in first complete remission. BMT may be superior to ABMT at least in second remission but here, too, data are inconclusive for firm recommendations.
Radiotherapy alone with extended or total lymphoid irradiation should be used in stage I large-cell NHL only if careful pathological staging can be carried out, while for stage II, combination chemotherapy should precede radiotherapy administration.
In lymphoblastic NHL a strategic approach similar to those employed in acute lymphoblastic leukaemia, i.e., with multidrug regimens with induction, consolidation and maintenance, prophylaxis of CNS relapse with intrathecal MTX and cranial irradiation has been shown as clearly superior to the conventional treatment of NHL [11-13]. Patients at high risk, i.e., with bone marrow or CNS involvement or elevated LDH at diagnosis, have a projected 5-year survival of less than 20%. These cases in first remission represent a suitable group to determine whether ABMT or BMT can improve survival.
Burkitt or Burkitt-like (small, non-cleaved) NHL requires a strategic approach which includes the use of one of the various intensive combinations similar to or derived from paediatric regimens [12-14]. Some authors suggest the initial use of debulking surgery or radiotherapy in an early phase of treatment with the aim of a better control of bulky disease. Combination chemotherapy should be administered as soon as possible. CNS prophylaxis is indicated [14].

Paediatric NHL

Survival of childhood NHL, although there are aggressive diffuse malignancies, has in the last 5 years increased to a point which, with the available drugs, probably cannot be improved upon. The desire of decreasing morbidity and sequelae should not deprive patients of a truly curative approach. This risk is obviously even higher for the patients with poor prognostic factors.

NHL in Elderly Patients (> 70 years)

Elderly patients who are in good general conditions (normal hepatic, cardiac and renal functions and high performance status) can tolerate standard combination chemotherapy (e.g., CHOP), but after 70 years only a minority of patients are judged eligible for intensive treatment. These patients more likely reveal alterations in kidney and liver function, and decreased bone marrow reserve with consequent higher morbidity [15]. The treatment decision should be based on the characteristics and conditions of the individual patient, not on the characteristic thought to be associated with age, until the results of prospective clinical trials on optimal treatment of elderly patients with NHL become available.

Peculiar Clinical Situations

- Meningeal involvement: methotrexate, and/or cytosine arabinoside, and prednisone should be administered intrathecally with concurrent cranial radiotherapy. Radiotherapy can be given as consolidation after CR induced by intrathecal chemotherapy.
- Gastrointestinal lymphomas: if feasible, gastrectomy, or resection of involved bowel segments, represent the best initial treatment, especially for patients with small-cell malignant lymphoma. Upfront combination chemotherapy carries the risk of visceral perforation [16]. In the case of resectable disease, it is not known whether subsequent chemotherapy provides an advantage compared to radiotherapy.
- Bulky disease: after CR to intensive combination chemotherapy, the use of radiotherapy is generally not advocated, while in patients who achieve PR radiotherapy could be necessary. For residual abdominal masses in aggressive NHL after combination chemotherapy, restaging laparotomy has a low yield [17]. Stable residual abdominal and mediastinal masses should only be closely followed.

- NHL patients with HIV infection: since the majority of these patients die because of rapid NHL progression, combination chemotherapy should be administered. Intensive combination chemotherapy can, however, only be delivered in patients with good performance status and absent or controlled opportunistic infections [18]. CHOP or CHOP-like combinations at reduced doses can be administered in patients with active opportunistic infections. Azidovudine should be administered concurrently with combination chemotherapy or as an alternative after achieving CR [18].

REFERENCES

1 Armitage JO and Cheson BD: Interpretation of clinical trials in diffuse large cell lymphomas. J Clin Oncol 1988 (6):1335-1347
2 NCI Hodgkin's Classification Project Writing Committee: Classification of non-Hodgkin's lymphomas: reproducibility of major classification systems. Cancer 1985 (55):91-95
3 Longo DL and De Vita VT: Malignant lymphomas. In: HM Pinedo and BA Chabner (eds) Cancer Chemotherapy Annual 8. Elsevier Science Publishers, Amsterdam 1986 pp 261-304
4 Coiffier B, Brousse N, Peuchmaur M, Berger F, Gisselbrecht C, Bryon PA, Diebold J: Peripheral T-cell lymphomas have a worse prognosis than B-cell lymphomas: a prospective study of 361 immunophenotyped patients treated with the LNH-84 regimen. Ann Oncol 1989 (1) in press
5 Klimo P and Connors JM: MACOP-B chemotherapy for the treatment of diffuse large-cell lymphomas. Ann Intern Med 1985 (102):596-602
6 Miller TP, Dahlberg S, Jones SE et al: ProMACE-CytaBOM is active with acceptable toxicity in patients with unfavourable non-Hodgkin lymphomas: a group-wide SWOG study. Proc Am Soc Clin Oncol 1987 (6):197
7 Longo D, De Vita V, Duffey PL et al: Randomized trial of ProMACE-MOPP vs Pro-MACE-CytaBOM in stage II-IV aggressive non-Hodgkin's lymphoma. Proc Am Soc Clin Oncol 1987 (6):206
8 Canellos GP, Skarin AT, Klatt MM et al: m-BACOP combination chemotherapy regimen in the treatment of diffuse large cell lymphoma. Semin Hematol 1981 (24):2-7
9 Coiffier B, Gisselbrecht C, Herbrecht R, Tilly H, Bosly A, Brousse N: LNH-84 regimen: a multicenter study on intensive chemotherapy in 737 patients with aggressive malignant lymphoma. J Clin Oncol 1989 (7):1018-1026
10 Coiffier B, Lepage E: Prognosis of aggressive lymphomas: a study of five prognostic models with patients included in the LNH-84 regimen. Blood 1989
11 Camitta BM, Lauer SJ, Casper JT, Kirchner PA, Kum LE, Oechler HW, Adair SE: Effectiveness of a six-drug regimen (APO) without local irradiation for treatment of mediastinal lymphoblastic lymphoma in children. Cancer 1985 (56):738-741
12 Amendola BE, Hutchinson R, Amendola MA, Schnitzer B: Childhood non-Hodgkin's lymphoma: a review of treatment results in 53 children. Eur Paediatr Haematol Oncol 1984 (1):213
13 Boguslawska-Jaworska J, Koscielnak E, Sroczynska M, Sonta-Jakimczyk, Armata J, Balwierz W, Ciepeilewska D, Kaczmarek-Kanold M, Ochocka M, Radwanska U, Rokicka-Milewska R: Evaluation of the LSA_2-L2 protocol for treatment of childhood non-Hodgkin's lymphoma. A report from the Polish Children's Leukemia/Lymphoma Study Group. Am J Pediatr Hematol Oncol 1984 (6):363-370
14 Sullivan MP, Ramirez I: Curability of Burkitt's lymphoma with high-dose cyclophosphamide-high-dose methotrexate therapy and intrathecal chemoprophilaxis. J Clin Oncol 1985 (3):627-636
15 Tirelli U, Zagonel V, Serraino D, Thomas J, Hoerni B, Tangury A, Ruhl U, Bey P, Tubiana N, Breed WPM, Roozendaal KJ, Hagenbeek A, Hupperets PS and Somers R: Non-Hodgkin's lymphomas in 137 patients aged 70 years or older: a retrospective European organization for research and treatment of cancer lymphoma group study. J Clin Oncol 1988 (6):1708-1713
16 Meyers PA, Potter VP, Wollner N, Exelby P: Bowel perforation during initial treatment for childhood non-Hodgkin's lymphoma. Cancer 1985 (56):259-261
17 Surbone A, Longo DL, De Vita VT, Ihde DC, Duffey PL, Jaffe ES, Solomon D, Hubbard SM and Young RC: Residual abdominal masses in aggressive non-Hodgkin's lymphoma after combination chemotherapy: significance and management. J Clin Oncol 1988 (6):1832-1837
18 Gisselbrecht C, Oksenhendler E, Farcet JP, Dombret H, Coiffier B, Thyss A, Raphael M: Treatment approaches for non-Hodgkin's lymphomas (NHL) associated with human immunodeficiency virus (HIV). Proc Am Soc Clin Oncol 1989 (8):3

GPSR Compliance

The European Union's (EU) General Product Safety Regulation (GPSR) is a set of rules that requires consumer products to be safe and our obligations to ensure this.

If you have any concerns about our products, you can contact us on ProductSafety@springernature.com

In case Publisher is established outside the EU, the EU authorized representative is:

Springer Nature Customer Service Center GmbH
Europaplatz 3
69115 Heidelberg, Germany

Batch number: 10684220

Printed by Printforce, the Netherlands